MENDEL'S GARDEN REVISITED
SELECTED MEDICAL TOPICS

David J. Holcombe

authorHOUSE®

AuthorHouse™
1663 Liberty Drive
Bloomington, IN 47403
www.authorhouse.com
Phone: 1 (800) 839-8640

Published by AuthorHouse 08/01/2018

ISBN: 978-1-5462-5317-4 (sc)
ISBN: 978-1-5462-5316-7 (e)

Cover design, "Portrait of Gregor Mendel" by Dr. David Holcombe

CONTENTS

ACKNOWLEDGEMENTS & DISCLAIMER

Medial topics become outdated almost before they are printed. These articles are no exception. Although there has been a sincere attempt to report the most current data, that information changes almost daily. At best, this collection is a snapshot in time, perhaps more of interest to sociologists and historians than to doctors or medical students.

Despite constant technological changes, certain themes remain constant over time and those, it is hoped, can be found throughout these pages. There has been no attempt to hide my personal liberal beliefs or profound sense of social justice. Both permeate these writings to a greater or lesser degree. Yet objectivity has no particular merit when changes in medicine and medical policy threaten the very fabric of our nation's health and well-being.

No specific cases are cited, except anecdotally, so there should be no HIPAA concerns. That being said, patients that are seen every day or every week cannot help but have an influence on the choice of topics and their treatment. My apologies to anyone who feels they have been personally targeted for their political beliefs or practice patterns. Also, although there are occasional references to other sources, this publication is written for the lay public and there is no attempt to provide comprehensive references for all information presented.

My thanks to the many patients, colleagues, collaborators and stakeholders who have helped shape these subjects and their interpretation. Most of these essays have appeared in CenLa Focus, a Central Louisiana publication that has solicited and published my observations over many years. The same is true of Visible Horizon, a publication of the Central Louisiana Council on Aging. Perhaps the latter fact explains the plethora of articles about the elderly.

My thanks to Dr. John Hill, who enjoyed proofreading the manuscript. If errors persist (which they always do), they are my fault, not his.

Although the articles are grouped under broad headings, their placement is sometimes arbitrary. Feel free to peruse the book in any order depending on your interest. Thank you, the reader, for taking the time to revisit Mendel's Garden.

PUBLIC HEALTH, AN INTRODUCTION: WHAT HAS IT DONE FOR YOU LATELY?

The general public has a poor understanding of what Public Health does and what it has accomplished. That confusion persists, especially among those over 50, because of the shifts in public health functions over the past decades. Older Louisianans, when asked, "What happens at the health units?" will invariable say "That's where kids get their shots." In fact, three decades ago, 88% of Louisianans did get their shots at a health unit, while now the number is closer to 10% or even less.

In Louisiana, public health has traditionally been associated with direct service care, notably immunizations, contraception, STD treatment and surveillance, and WIC (Women, Infants and Children) food supplementation programs. While direct care by public health still serves as a safety net for some services, there are other states that adhere to the core public health functions (i.e. surveillance, connecting people with services, dissemination of information, enforcement of regulations, development of policies, research and creating a competent public health work force). Providing direct care when no other providers are available (notably for contraception and STD treatment) remains a part of public health, as in Louisiana, but not a core function in many parts of the U.S.

So what has public health nationally done for our country? Those accomplishments include 10 activities most people will recognize:

1. Reducing disease through vaccine use remains a triumph. There has been huge decreases in all "vaccine preventable disease," more recently rotavirus, meningococcus, pneumococcal pneumonia, as well as the other childhood diseases: measles, mumps, rubella,

polio, diphtheria, whooping cough, chickenpox and hepatitis, both A and B. Many of these diseases are so rare now that patients (and even doctors) have never seen them. Failure to vaccinate, however, carries with it enormous negative consequences, underestimated by the "anti-vaccinators."

2. Prevention and control of infectious diseases through screening, surveillance and treatment, notably with TB and HIV, have resulted in huge improvements in survival through timely treatment.

3. Promotion of tobacco control with increases of tobacco taxes, proliferation of smoke-free ordinances at local and state levels, restricted advertising and aggressive education campaigns, have resulted in a decrease in tobacco use nationally from 42% of adults in 1965 to 20% or less now. Any reduction in tobacco use saves lives.

4. Improving maternal and infant health through the mandated use of folic acid in grains, and the generalized use of neonatal screening for a host of treatable infant disorders have reduced cases of spina bifida and resulted in earlier diagnosis and treatment of many genetic disorders.

5. Enhancing motor vehicle safety through mandated seatbelt and child safety seat use and, improving safety by promoting changes in the road construction and signage have resulted in steady declines in motor vehicle death rates.

6. Reducing cardiovascular death by promoting and standardizing treatment for hypertension, cholesterol and tobacco cessation has saved millions of lives.

7. Occupational safety promotion using best practices, notably for lifting and use of farm equipment (especially for children), has reduced injuries and workman's compensation cases.

8. Increasing cancer screenings to improve survival following early diagnosis, especially in breast cancer and colon caner has resulted in improved survival rates.

9. Aggressive screening programs have reduced lead poisoning from 88.2% of high-risk children in 2003 to less than 1% in 2008 (notably in African-American children in substandard housing.)

10. Development of national and state emergency response systems with the use of the National Incident Management System and improvement in the coordination of state and local resources produced remarkable results in the responses to Hurricanes Gustav, Ike, Isaac and Harvey in Louisiana (and other emergencies nationally.)

Public health, as enigmatic as it sounds, continues to play a role in communities throughout Louisiana and the U.S. The safety net function of their services depends on the availability of local providers, but the other core functions will remain, regardless of those circumstances. The collaborations and cooperative efforts generated by public health go a long way in promoting healthier communities even though those efforts may not always be evident. Whether it's a public health nurse, sanitarian, nutritionist, disease intervention or surveillance specialist or the Regional Administrator, feel free to give them a call. They have a wealth of information and experience and a willingness to share both.

BEHAVIORAL HEALTH

RETIREMENT, I'LL DRINK TO THAT! OR BETTER NOT!

Although many people look forward to the pleasures of retirement, the reality may be worse than anticipated. Thirty-five million people in the U.S. are 65 or older with the number increasing daily. Many seniors will reach retirement age whether they want it or not. While some people choose to retire, others will be forced into retirement by medical conditions, layoffs or competition with younger employees.

Once retired, seniors may find themselves with a sense of purposelessness, isolation, economic stains, relational changes and depression. Many will seek solace in substance abuse, notably with alcohol. It is estimated that around three million Americans over 55 years of age abuse alcohol and that number may rise to over 6 million by 2020. Besides the numerous health-related issues such as cirrhosis, neuropathy and dementia associated with alcohol, increased instability results in more slips and falls with associated fractures. In an article in "Work, Aging and Retirement," Dr. Bamberger states that health problems related to alcohol has cost over 60 billion dollars in hospital-related costs in the 1990's. This includes $300 million for addiction treatment.

While alcohol is the most common substance abused, benzodiazepines and pain relievers are often involved. Such combinations only increase risks to the elderly. Unfortunately, many seniors, their families and even their physicians fail to recognize substance abuse. Doctors recognize substance abuse in younger patients 67% of the time, but only 37% of the time in the elderly.

Use of brief screening tools (such as SBIRT) helps increase diagnosis, but awareness alone does not necessarily translate into change. Seniors need access to effective addiction programs that take their unique medical challenges into consideration. Family members need to be vigilante for increased instability, confusion, isolation or depression, all of which may be signs of alcohol use (or other medical conditions). Both the senior and their entourage should accept the possibility of an substance abuse and seek treatment.

Those nearing retirement need to anticipate economic and emotional changes. Family, friends and other support systems play a critical role. Volunteerism may also play a positive role. Louisiana has a very low rate of senior volunteerism, though opportunities exist through churches, civic organizations, libraries, museums and other venues. States with high senior volunteer rates also have corresponding better results for senior health. Perhaps there is not a direct cause and effect relationship, but senior volunteerism is good for the senior and the community.

Retirement may be the end of one phase of life, but it can be the beginning of another in which relevance and social engagement still play important roles. Substance abuse, whether it is with alcohol or legal drugs is a problem. If you must "drink to retirement," save if for the retirement party and consider a non-alcoholic beverage.

BINGE DRINKING IN WOMEN

Binge drinking is periodic excessive consumption of alcohol in excess of the recommended limit of one glass of wine or two beers a day. While generally associated with men, binge drinking has become a problem in women as well. One in eight women engages in binge drinking, as do one in five high school girls (less than 18 years old). Binging usually entails the consumption of 6 alcoholic drinks per episode, which occurs 3 times a month or more.

Binge drinking kills around 23,000 girls and women each year. When done during pregnancy, it can result in fetal deformity or death. Binge drinking also increased a woman's risk for breast cancer, heart disease, STDs, and unintended pregnancies. Excessive episodic alcohol consumption leads to increased injuries (fall, MVAs and drowning) and can lead to chronic alcoholism in some cases. Long-term binging is also associated with increased domestic violence, including assaults and homicides. Long-term health risks include hypertension, coronary artery disease, stroke and cirrhosis.

Binge drinkers are also more likely to engage in drunk driving, something in which Louisiana exceeds the national average. Over 3,000 Louisianans of both sexes died from accidents involving drunk driving from 2003 to 2012. While more men died than women, the latter still had a death rate of 2.4/100,000 in Louisiana, double the national rate for women (1.2/100.000).

Binging varies with age, but occurs at all ages in women. About 20% of high school girls binge drink. This increases to 24% of women in the 18-24 age range and dips down slightly to 20% in women 25 to 34. After that, it drops to only 15% of women from 35 to 44 and drops to only 10% in women 45 to 64. Only 3% of women over 65 years of age binge drink.

During high school, alcohol use (not necessarily binge drinking) increases from 45% of freshman to 65% of seniors. A third of these girls will binge drink. White women binge drink more than African-American and Hispanic women although the difference evens out with age (when only 10-13% of adult women binge.)

The first step toward a solution is recognizing the breadth and depth of the problem. Women should limit alcohol consumption to one drink per day. No alcohol is safe during pregnancy when it poses a health risk to both mother and fetus. Direct marketing of alcohol to youth should be eliminated and age-related restrictions should be enforced.

Healthcare workers and caregivers should always ask about alcohol consumption both in men and women and discuss the short and long-term risks of binging. While most women bingers are not alcoholics, professional counseling may be necessary in some cases. Since adolescents are at risk for all high-risk behaviors, they should be targeted for education, role-playing and, in cooperation with parents, avoiding high-risk situations where alcohol is consumed.

ALZHEIMER'S DISEASE AND BENZODIAZEPINES: A SMOKING GUN?

Alzheimer's disease has been called the "silent epidemic." In the United States alone, there are over 5 million Alzheimer's sufferers (most of them women), a third of whom will die from their disease. An army of 15.5 million caregivers devotes 17.7 billion hours of unpaid assistance annually, amounting to $220 billion dollars. Worldwide, it has been estimated that there are over 36 million people who suffer from the disease, a number that will double every 20 years, reaching over 115 million by 2050.

Benzodiazepines are a popular class of medication used for anxiety and insomnia. Some of the more familiar and widely used products include alprazolam (Xanax®), lorazepam (Ativan®), diazepam (Valium®), all three used for anxiety, and flurazepam (Dalmane®), temazepam (Restoril®) and triazolam (Halcion®) used for sleep. Diazepam (Valium®), released in 1963, remained one of the best-selling medications from 1969 to 1982 in the U.S. In 2002, 13.7% of all Medicare beneficiaries received some form of benzodiazepine. Those with chronic mental illness, younger Medicare beneficiaries, women and those with lower incomes were disproportionately represented among the recipients.

Although benzodiazepines are ideally recommended for short courses of therapy (1-2 weeks to three months at most), longer term use often occurs, resulting in habituation or frank addition. It is well known that benzodiazepines increase instability among the elderly, resulting in increased falls and other accidents. The American Geriatrics Society listed benzodiazepines among those drugs considered "potentially inappropriate for seniors because of risks like confusion, dizziness and falls."

More recently, an article in the British Medical Journal explored the possibility that benzodiazepines also increase the risk of Alzheimer's disease. Around 9,000 seniors in Quebec Province were studied and the results showed an increase of Alzheimer's disease from 43-51% among benzodiazepine users. Not surprisingly, the longer the exposure, the greater the risk, which was also increased with longer acting benzodiazepines.

The authors did concede that early manifestations of Alzheimer's might result in increased symptoms of anxiety and insomnia, which were subsequently treated with benzodiazepines. Nonetheless, they concluded that physicians must "comply with good practice guidelines-that is, the shortest duration with a preference for formulations with a short half-life." The basic tenant of medicine still remains *"primum non nocere"* (first and foremost, do no harm). Let us not contribute to the advancing avalanche of Alzheimer's patients. Implement "good practice guidelines" and limit long-term use, especially of long-acting benzodiazepines.

Billioti de Gage, S, Y Moride, T Ducruet et al. Benzodiazipine use and risk of Alzheimer's disease: case-control study. BMJ 2014: 349:g5205

OPIOID ABUSE: A NATIONAL EPIDEMIC

Abuse of opioids (narcotic pain relievers) in the U.S. has increased four times over the last decade (1990's). Deaths from opioid pain relievers have simultaneously increased at the same rate. While states vary in their statistics, Louisiana ranks among the higher states for opioid use and among the highest for opioid-related deaths. Over 5% of adult Louisianans (over 225,000) engage in NON-medical use of opioids, resulting in 15 deaths/100,000 residents (or around 675 deaths a year). Sales of opioids amount to 6.8 kilograms (15 lbs.)/100,000 Louisiana residents per year.

The extent of the problem is staggering since deaths are only the tip of the iceberg. For every opioid-related death, there are 32 emergency room visits for overdose, 136 people who are addicted and 825 NON-medical opioid users. For Louisiana, this translates into 21,000 ER visits, 92,000 opioid addicts and 555,000 non-medical users (or about 12% of the state's population or the equivalent of the entire population of Jefferson Parish).

With crackdowns on the illegal use of prescription opioids, there has been a corresponding increase in heroin use. Law enforcement personnel have likened this phenomenon to "Whack-a-mole," where creative addicts and entrepreneurs find alternative sources when one dries up or becomes too expensive. Florida noticed that when Oxycontin® diversion (illegal use) through "pill mills" decreased, legal methadone use increased proportionally and parallel to illegal use of heroin.

Where does this torrent of opioids come from? Among users, over half of it is provided at no cost from well-meaning friends and relatives who "share" their pain medications. Doctors prescribe about 18%, while another 16% is stolen or purchased from family members or friends. Drug dealers account for 4% and Internet purchases make up another 1%. These proportions change with long-term addiction, which shifts to increased illegal sources. Risk factors for slipping from legitimate use into abuse are (1) prior history of substance abuse, (2) underlying psychiatric disorders, (3) younger age (adolescents) and (4) a family history of substance abuse. Length of use also plays an important role.

Although non-narcotic pain relievers should always be the first treatment option, they can and do fail to relieve some chronic pain. Prescription of narcotics remains a constant challenge to all physicians and hesitancy must not be construed as a lack of compassion, but rather the wisdom born out of difficult therapeutic experiences with substance abusers. Current recommendations have also changed for all professional organizations with respect to opioid prescriptions.

What should the patient expect with long-term use of extended release or long-acting opioids? First, the physician, usually a pain specialist, will expect complete prior medical records from the patient. Second, you must undergo a thorough medical exam, including a urine drug test (which will be repeated periodically.) Third, you will fill out an "Opioid Risk Tool" or some other similar document to assess your susceptibility to substance abuse. Fourth, physicians will consult the Prescription Monitoring Program, run by the LA Board of Pharmacy, that tracks all narcotic prescriptions by all providers in order to reveal "doctor shopping."

Goals of therapy will be to (1) decrease pain, (2) restore function and (3) improve the secondary consequences of pain (i.e. weakness, instability, and maladaptive behavior). Before initiation of Extended Release (ER) or Long Acting (LA) Opioids, you will also be expected to fill out a "Patient Prescriber Agreement," a document explaining risks and benefits and outlying patient policies and expectations. Dosing of ER/LA opioids is complex and requires considerable expertise, especially when changes are made due to the variety of available medications and their different pharmacodynamics.

Despite all of the precautions, patients may intentionally or unintentionally overdose, resulting in respiratory depression and death. Given the increase in deaths associated with increased heroin use, the FDA approved a new automatic naloxone injector (Evzio®). A newer, much cheaper generic version now exists as well and can be obtained without a prescription in many states. Naloxone (Narcan®) reverses the opioid effects and may prove lifesaving. The injector can be administered directly through clothing into the lateral aspect (side) of the upper thigh. The generic version can be administered in an easy-to-use nasal spray. Naloxone use is not intended to substitute for an emergency room visit, which should follow any episode for respiratory failure.

Opioids have transformed the lives of chronic pain sufferers, but they must be used appropriately and prescribed by trained professionals. Unfortunately, opioid use and abuse has multiplied in the last decades and has become a problem of catastrophic proportions, prompting President Trump to declare a national health emergency. All providers and patients should be part of the solution and not part of the problem. Never use opioids as a first choice pain reliever, start low and go slow if you must use an opioid, monitor prior to and during use and remember "primum non nocere" (first and foremost, do no harm).

SCLEROSIS, A DANGER FOR INDIVIDUALS AND INSTITUTIONS

Older individuals have been bombarded with recommendations to avoid sclerosis (loss of flexibility or "hardening"), whether it is intellectual or physical. The danger for individuals of loss of flexibility also holds true for collective bodies. Hierarchical institutions, whether they are academic, charitable, for-profit or governmental, all become susceptible to sclerosis through three mechanisms: (1) the "Peter Principle," (2) distancing from the field, and (3) "groupthink." These concepts are not new, but their recognition and vigilance in preventing them should be a personal and institutional priority.

(1) As groups become bigger and more hierarchical, several things occur. There is the well-known phenomenon of the "Peter Principle," which states that individuals rise in an organization until they become increasingly incompetent (unable to master their expanded role and responsibilities.) While these same individuals were well adapted and functional at a lower organizational level, this advantage can evaporate as they rise in positions requiring new and different skill sets. This can result in marginally competent individuals in high places.

(2) Another related phenomenon occurs when knowledge of, understanding of, and sympathy for those working in distant field operations becomes more tenuous as organizations expand and individuals rise in the hierarchy. Although this need not occur, especially in those who have "come from the field," the responsibilities and preoccupations related to upper management can blind those in higher positions to the day-to-day realities of the business "on the ground," whatever it may be. This can

lead to decisions that are counter-productive to field operations with little incentive to make necessary corrections.

(3) The so-called "group think" phenomena appears related to both the "Peter Principle" (rising to one's highest level of incompetence) and distancing from the field. It represents an unhealthy manifestation of what Robert Putnam called "bonding social capital" (or coming together of people with similar views, lifestyles, looks and incomes.) As individuals rise in the hierarchy, their preoccupations turn more toward maintaining and enhancing their power and compensation rather than caring for the health and growth of the organization they govern and the people they serve.

Group think members can become absorbed with personal agendas, unrelated to the organizational mission, as they gradually weed out those people who do not share their thinking. Members of the "inner group" become progressively more rigid, paranoid and unwilling to accept dissent or diversity. What might have begun as collegiality among a leadership group with "bonding social capital," can coalesce into a sinister and vindictive unit with narrow personal goals, associated with an abundance of shifting personal alliances. Organizations infected with groupthink become rigid, unresponsive and progressively out of touch with their clients, both external or internal (field personnel).

Whether the organization is a for-profit business, a not-for-profit, a church or governmental entity, the dangers of institutional sclerosis remain the same. Brittle, self-serving administrations cannot adapt to change, especially since they stifle creativity and dissent. They guarantee a loss of flexibility, indispensable for long-term institutional adaptability and survival.

Antidotes to sclerosis for individuals involve physical and mental exercise to maintain agility. For individuals and groups, the antidote also involves what Robert Putnam calls the cultivation of "bridging social capital." This latter is characterized by leadership creating groups that contain a wide diversity of people with different incomes, life-styles, races and backgrounds. Healthy organizations foster a culture of inclusiveness, which tolerates and rewards the "other" rather than excluding them through fear and self-interest. Positive inclusion results in an increased opportunity for long-term personal and institutional survival.

Efforts to increase "bridging social capital" require vision and leadership, not always recognized or encouraged in large institutional settings. Long-term benefits for health, however, for both individuals and institutions become an inevitable byproduct of such a positive orientation. As individuals or groups, we should be on the lookout for ways to enhance bridging social capital, so easy to understand in theory and so difficult to achieve in real life.

NARCISSISTIC ENTITLEMENT SYNDROME AND THE FOUNDER'S COMPLEX: TWO INTERESTING PSYCHOLOGICAL PROFILES

Any work environment can be fraught with psychological pitfalls. While most office conflicts can be overcome with some goodwill and sustained communication, two psychological profiles can result in serious consequences for any organization.

The first is the Narcissistic Entitlement Syndrome (NES). It derives its name from the famous Greek myth in which Narcissus falls in love with his own reflection and pines away with unrequited love. Out of pity, the gods transformed him into a flower that grows near ponds and often hangs over the water's edge where it is mirrored in the still water below.

Sufferers of the Narcissistic Entitlement Syndrome have a disproportionate sense of their own special skills and contributions. They become excessively demanding, often at the expense of others around them. Although it is more common in younger workers, it can affect any age group. Estimates put this personality type at 10% of any workforce.

Such individuals remain self-serving and oblivious of the needs of those around them. They feel a sense of fully justified entitlement to special treatment or privileges due to their supposed unusual intelligence, abilities, qualifications or past success. Although everyone fantasizes about their own powers, those with NES are obsessed with them, projecting an arrogant attitude to others. They project disdain for the common folk around them and seek out others they perceive as sharing their distinctive abilities.

They solicit constant approval and admiration and react with rage at any real or perceived criticism. Lacking empathy, they also quickly become envious of others who may be succeeding. Those with NES tend to gradually find themselves bitter and isolated, often changing jobs and friendships in a vain hope of finding the perfect environment for their distinctive talents.

The Founder's Complex entails some of the same negative attributes of NES, although it may be found in individuals with true talent and ability. In the Founder's Complex, the individual is totally psychologically invested in a project or organization of their creation. As founder, they feel that no one else has the ability or talent to take over their dominant role.

The founder will often denigrate or sabotage those seeking to assure succession, jealously guarding their power. They may even prefer to see their organization or project cease to exist rather than see it pass into the hands of those whom they perceive as unworthy or incompetent. In that respect, they share some of the traits of arrogance and lack of empathy that characterize those with the Narcissistic Entitlement Syndrome.

Where the two differ is that the founder demonstrates true organizational ability where the person with NES exaggerates their own abilities. But the founder lacks the vision and imagination to see others as capable of assuming the leadership position. Their project is their baby and the baby must die rather than fall into the hands of other unqualified and less deserving parents.

Whether a person is narcissistic with a defective image of self or a founder with a true sense of their own ability, both lack a fundamental sense of the value of others, except as a means to their ends. The adulation both crave blinds them to the needs of others and makes true collaboration in the workplace extremely difficult.

Both of these profile types should be approached with caution since their intelligence, often extreme, makes them dangerous adversaries. If they are your employees, beware of their destructive influence on others, if they are your bosses, you can stay and suffer or choose to leave. Changing either personality type, especially if they are older, is a daunting task at best, impossible at worst.

SOCIAL SUPPORT AND
ALL-CAUSE MORTALITY

Intuitively, most people would assume that sociable people might live longer than curmudgeonly, isolated ones. Katie Becovsky and her colleagues at the Mayo Clinic studied the question. They followed 3220 patients (25% of them women) from 1990 to 2003 or until the subject's death. The average age of participants at the beginning of the study was 53 years old, with the youngest being in their 40's and the oldest in their 60's. They evaluated the amount of social support that subjects received from their spouses or partners, relatives and friends with whom they had regular contact.

Perhaps not surprisingly, they found that social support from a spouse, partner and close relatives, combined with weekly interactions with from 6 to 7 friends, resulted in reduced risk of death. While such factors as diet, physical activity and tobacco use have been well established in relation to longevity, the role of social contacts has not been closely studied.

Becovsky et al. speculated that some companionship can also be obtained from pet ownership, which may increase physical activity and also provide needed "social support." Yet the fact remains that interacting with other people has a protective effect on health. Unfortunately, illness and our car-oriented society greatly decrease the opportunity for some individuals, especially the elderly, to interact with others. Older cities and villages were often designed prior to the advent of automobiles and maintain pedestrian friendly dimensions. Not so our modern suburban designs in which there may be no sidewalks, no crosswalks on busy streets, no readily accessible supermarkets or other stores. Since the elderly may lack the ability or the confidence to drive, they may become socially isolated, reducing their interpersonal contacts and increasing their all-cause mortality.

Jeff Anderson has suggested the following to reduce social isolation: (1) Provide transportation to the elderly, (2) Encourage volunteerism, (3) Promote worship, (4) Have a pet, (5) Boost senior self-esteem, (6) Optimize vision and hearing, (7) Invest in "adaptive technologies" (i.e. walkers, ramps, safety bars), (8) Be an attentive neighbor, (9) Eat in a group, (10) Address incontinence, (11) Hug a senior, (12) Recognize and treat depression, especially resulting from grieving, (13) Find a caring physician, attentive to the elderly and (14) Support caregivers. Mr. Anderson's list provides a number of simple ways to address the issue of elderly isolation. We all need to be part of the social network that helps keep the elderly engaged and healthy. Isolation increases the risk for death. Let's not be a contributing part of the all-cause mortality.

Becofsky, KM et al. Influence of the Source of Social Support and Size of Social Network on All-Cause Mortality. *Mayo Clin Proc*. July 2015:90(7):895-902.

STRESS AND THE ELDERLY

As has often been said, getting old is not for the faint of heart. With aging comes a host of stressors including deteriorating health, financial worries, deaths of a spouse or other loved ones, adjustments to retirement, loss of independence and worries about your own death. Reactions to stress, at least when it is acute in nature, include our "fight or fight" responses. We have a surge of adrenaline and cortisol, both of which help us deal with the immediate crisis. Unfortunately, most of the stresses facing the elderly are more chronic and repetitive in nature and so are their deleterious effects.

Emotional responses to stress can include anxiety, fear, restlessness, poor concentration, forgetfulness and depression. In fact, the spectrum of psychiatric responses to stress in aging can and do include a host of disorders: Acute stress disorder, post-traumatic stress disorder, panic attacks, social anxiety, generalized anxiety disorder (GAD), depression and, less often, phobias and obsessive-compulsive disorder. It is estimated that 10% of adults 55 to 85 years old suffer from anxiety disorder, about the same percentage as in other age groups.

Some of the physiological responses to stress may include loss of appetite, insomnia, muscle aches and pains, palpitations, urinary frequency and generalized fatigue. Other long-term physiological responses result in a combination of increased risks for cardiovascular disease, high blood pressure, sleep disorders, irritable bowel syndrome and stress ulcers. The same chronic stress spills over to care givers, many of whom suffer with mental and physical disorders, with the same devastating consequences.

As Richard Carlson put it, "Stress is nothing more than a socially acceptable form of mental illness." That being said, what are the potential solutions? First, recognition is primary for prevention. Understanding that the issues of loss of control and independence, deteriorating physical and psychological conditions, and the trauma associated with retirement or the loss of loved ones, are all going to precipitate stress and some sort of stress response, either appropriate or exaggerated.

Second, some positive factors can temper inappropriate responses. Maintaining an active physical and mental existence helps keep the body and mind agile, adaptable and occupied. Being active with grandchildren and other family and social groups (such as faith-based organizations) provides restorative interactions and counters a tendency for withdrawal and isolation. Older people, especially through volunteerism, can be valued for their knowledge and wisdom. Third, recognizing one's own continuing contributions and accomplishments helps maintain a positive attitude and enhances a contagious self-esteem.

When the responses to the stress of aging become pathological, professional assistance should be obtained. This is especially true when self-medication with alcohol or other substances are involved. There are also professional techniques of biofeedback, acupuncture and yoga that can prove helpful. (Although, as an anonymous wit once declared, "I've tried yoga, but I find stress less boring.")

Maintaining an active life will perhaps allow you to say what Henry Kissinger once said, "There cannot be a stressful crisis next week. My schedule is already full."

PHYSICIAN BURNOUT: A COSTLY AND DANGEROUS PROBLEM

Physician burnout was first described by Herbert Freudenberger in the 1970's in his book "Burnout: The High Cost of High Achievement." It was subsequently identified as an occupational hazard in health care professionals. A study in 2011 identified 38% of physicians that suffer from burnout, a percentage that rose to 40% in 2013 and 51% in 2017. Those specialists at higher risk were emergency medicine (59%), OB/GYN (56%), followed by family medicine, internal medicine and infectious diseases (55%). Although some specialties appeared less subject to burnout (i.e. dermatology, otolaryngology and ophthalmology) all specialties had some manifestations. Burnout appears to also vary with the ethnicity of physicians with Asian Indians (46%) suffering the least and Chinese (56%) the most, with Whites, Filipino and African-Americans all in between (around 50%).

The causes of burnout include bureaucratic burdens, mostly related to the requirements of electronic health records and regulatory requirements, including "click fatigue" and "alert fatigue." However, there were emotional issues, too, which include prolonged working hours, stressful decision making, worry, a loss of meaning in the profession and a generally poor work/life balance. Since over 60% of doctors are now women, the latter has become particularly important. Almost no one claimed to be "extremely happy," especially among those who reported high levels of burnout. Other causes of concern included the dehumanization of their position, loss of autonomy, and the omnipresent danger of litigation with its corrosive effect on the physician-patient relationship. The leadership qualities of a doctor's supervisor also play a critical role. There must be some true caring that recognizes physicians for a job well done and empowers and inspires them to continue.

Since few people have sympathy for highly paid professionals, you may wonder why this is important to the general public. In fact, physician burnout turns out to be a dangerous and costly problem. Burnout results in early retirement, reductions in work time, and turnover of employed physicians, fatigue and distractions with resulting unnecessary testing, referrals and even prescriptions for antibiotics. Physician errors increase and with them an increased risk for malpractice, with its litany of additional stressors for the clinician. One large health care system estimated that it cost around $750,000 to recruit and train new physicians, not to mention the costs of lost revenue. Predictably, doctors suffering from burnout are prone to depression, divorce, and 400 will take their own lives every year.

It has taken time for the health care community to wake up to this expensive and dangerous problem. Medical schools have established wellness programs to provide emotional and physical support. There are efforts to re-build trust and collegial bonds between doctors, who may view each other more as competitors than trusted colleagues. Efforts are being made to make electronic health records more user friendly. Institutional leaders must recognize the issues and recognize the complicity of their organization in physician burnout. Measures of well-being among providers need to be evaluated as well as the leadership qualities of the administration. Turnover, early retirement, job slowdowns and overt depression must be addressed promptly and with sincerity. Collaborative teams need to be encouraged, and every attempt made to recognize and address the burden of electronic health records.

The tragedy of the American malpractice system also needs to be addressed. Once sued, doctors are discouraged or forbidden to seek support from colleagues and friends. This only aggravates what can be a long, painful and discouraging process, regardless of the outcome. Forced arbitration and the elimination of contingency-based legal fees would provide immeasurable relief to a system destructive system to all but the plaintiff's attorneys.

Burnout is a system failure, not an individual one. While patients deserve a competent and compassionate workforce, physicians need to recognize their own humanity and the institutions they work for must do the same. More of the same will result in deteriorating quality, physician depression, a lost or broken work force and even in the suicide of some providers. Surely we cannot afford to sacrifice such valuable members of our society to the ravages of physician burnout.

CHRONIC DISEASES AND CANCER

BREAST CANCER: THE INSIDIOUS ENEMY

Despite billions of dollars of research and treatment, breast cancer remains a leading killer of women. In 2015 and the years beyond, it is estimated that there will be 200,000 new cases of breast cancer and 40,000 women will die from the disease during the year. Even though awareness, screening and treatment have undergone tremendous improvements over the last decade, almost everyone still knows a friend, family member or acquaintance who has died from breast cancer. Why does breast cancer refuse to go away? And why do women continue to die from this terrible killer?

First, breast cancer is not one entity, but many. There is considerable diversity among breast cancers with respect to their specific histological forms, genetic makeup, hormonal sensitivities, responsiveness to treatment and outcomes.

Second, women (and men) who suffer from breast cancer are as different as the many variations of the disease itself. Genetic susceptibility varies greatly as does the propensity to develop breast cancer based on risk factors such as obesity and a history of no breast-feeding. There are also individual variations in response to standardized treatment based on genetics, other familial characteristics and pre-existing medical conditions.

Third, while breast cancer survival depends on the stage at diagnosis (the earlier the better) that remains an oversimplification. Sadly, at all stages of diagnosis, with all women, survival from breast cancer also depends on your insurance status. Privately insured women (and men) do better and survive longer than those with no insurance or those with Medicaid (the two latter survival curves being almost identical.) (This finding also holds true for colon cancer survival, for which your survival also depends, to a major extent, on your insurance status.) Although that may seem intuitive, the fact remains that patients with no insurance or Medicaid are predominately poor and African-American and Hispanic and suffer the worst outcomes. The American Cancer Society publicized this disturbing finding several years ago. The implications of these revelations are that eliminating disparities between those treated with private insurance and those with Medicaid or without insurance would help improve breast cancer survival significantly in these latter groups. Disparities can be attributed to the social determinants of income, educational level and social status, all very difficult to improve.

Last, but not least, breast cancer is truly an insidious enemy with an almost unique profile. While many cancer victims (such as those with early resectable colon cancer) are considered "cured" if they reach the 5-year disease free survival point, breast cancer has no such guarantees. As a local surgeon, Dr. David McCoy, pointed out, breast cancer is not an organ-specific disease, but rather a "systemic disease." Many women, correctly and aggressively treated for their breast cancer will sail past their 5-year mark only to be diagnosed with widespread disease at 10 or even 15 years post treatment. This disheartening reality devastates the victims and their family, friends and medical providers.

Given the variability of the disease, the diversity of the hosts, the vagaries of insurance and the insidious nature of breast cancer itself, what can be done? Research certainly has improved diagnosis and treatment, with more customized approaches to each patient, and will likely continue to do so. Universal screening with mammograms at the appropriate ages must still occur. The controversies surrounding the optimal time to initiate mammograms (whether it be 40, 45 or 50) still confuses the public and professionals alike. That being said, any woman, at any age, who detects a breast mass should seek professional help. No one should wait beyond 50 years of age for her first screening mammogram.

Exploding costs for cancer treatments also complicate the situation. Realistic approaches with cost/benefit ratios must guide those involved with individual treatment options. It does little good to add a few weeks or months to a patient's life when the process may bankrupt the patient and their grieving family. As painful as it is, demand will always remain unlimited and resources will always be limited. Policy makers, insurers, providers and the general public must work together to achieve realistic goals while tempering unrealistic expectations. Our common insidious enemy, breast cancer, still remains to be defeated.

Recently, Governor John Bel Edwards and the Secretary of Health, Dr. Rebekah Gee, have proposed a new cooperative approach to cancer in Louisiana among patients, providers and payers.

BREAST CANCER SCREENING AND THE PROMISE OF GENOMICS

Controversy continues to surround the optimal time to initiate screening mammograms. Diagnostic mammograms (unlike screening mammograms) can be started at any age since they are used to "diagnose" palpable masses or other abnormal masses or lesions discovered on exam. But true screening mammograms (in the absence of a palpable mass) continue to pose a particular dilemma.

The United States Preventive Task Force (USPTS) recommends starting screening mammograms at age 50. As a layperson, you might think "the sooner the better," but, in fact, early screening mammograms may reveal lesions that, after further investigations (up to and including biopsy), are found to be "false positives." False positives (as opposed to true positives) are when the screening test appears positive, but no malignancy is identified with a biopsy. The added worry, testing and expense do not, according to the USPTF, justify screening earlier than age 50 and only result in rampant over-diagnosis, which may represent from 14.7 to 25% of all screen-detected lesions.

In contrast, the American Cancer Society and some other organizations still recommend starting annual screening mammograms at age 45, going to biannual after 55 years old. They contend that earlier diagnosis does justify earlier screening and that women should have the right to request screening mammograms as early as 40. Despite false positives (and the additional worry, side effects and cost of additional tests), earlier diagnoses do increase survival for certain women with certain types of breast cancers, but not for all women. The goal of screening, of course, is to save lives. The theory is that the earlier the diagnosis, the earlier the stage and the better the treatment options and survival.

Unfortunately, other factors such as insurance status further complicates the issue of outcomes. Women with private insurance demonstrate significantly higher 5 years survival than women who are either uninsured or have Medicaid. Those issues mostly revolve around social determinants related to poverty, low education and low social status. To further complicate outcomes, breast cancer occurs in a host of variants related to cell type, hormone sensitivity and other traits related to their genetic make up.

Genetic mapping of breast cancers (genomics) has proven to be a boon to scientist's and oncologists. Whereas formerly most breast cancers were treated in a similar way (with variations of surgical resection, radiation and chemotherapy, depending on the type of cancer), it has become possible through genomics to identify breast tumors that only require tumorectomy and no other complimentary therapies. Results for such tumors remain excellent and spare women from needless expense and side effects due to unnecessary treatments. Genomics also helps identify tumors that will respond better to specific chemotherapy that can be tailored more specifically to the type of tumor. Some tumors do not represent a clinical threat at all and can be safely observed.

While breast cancer survival has improved over time, it remains a deadly foe, killing 40,000 U.S. women a year. Sadly, it can also sometimes recur ten, fifteen or twenty years after an apparent cure, a demoralizing fact for patients and doctors alike. Screening, treatment and prognostic indicators do, however, continue to evolve. We now have breast CAT scans, 3-dimineitional mammography, stereotactic biopsies and genomics. But while scientific progress will surely continue to occur, we must also address the social determinants of poverty, poor education and low social status that have proven just as tenacious as breast cancer itself and just as deadly.

Whatever your age, you and your doctor need to decide together when to start screening, just be sure and get your mammogram.

COLORECTAL CANCER: STILL A PROBLEM

Colorectal cancer remains a significant problem in Louisiana. Even though we have a highly effective screening method (i.e. colonoscopy), only 64.3% of adults over 50 have been screened. The inevitable result of low screening is a high number of new cases of colorectal cancer in Louisiana (3rd in the U.S.) and the 4th highest mortality rate among states.

Louisiana's 5 year incidence rate for colorectal (new cases) is 92.9/100,000 Louisianans, significantly higher than the 70.8/100,000 nationally. As with most cancers, the earlier the diagnosis, the better the outcomes (and the lower the 5 year mortality). Since many Louisianans are diagnosed in late stages (over half in Stage III or Stage IV, regional or distant metastases respectively), death rates are correspondingly higher.

The other sad reality is that death rates are higher depending on your insurance status, with lower survivals among those with Medicaid or who are completely uninsured compared to those with other insurance. Since African-Americans are over-represented among Medicaid recipients and the uninsured, their death rates remain higher than with Whites (an example of so-called health disparities) and characteristic of other cancers in Louisiana: breast, prostate and lung.

The Louisiana Colorectal Cancer Roundtable is a collaboration among insurers and providers with a goal of increasing the screening rates from the current 64.3% up to 80% or higher. By so doing, we could eliminate 3,471 deaths due to colorectal cancer annually and save at least some of the over $350 million spent on this avoidable disease. If 80% colorectal cancer screening could be achieved, 277,000 new cases would be averted and over 200,000 lives could be saved within 20 years. Governor John Bel Edwards and Dr. Rebekah Gee, Secretary of Health for the Louisiana Department of Health, have recently launched an updated version of the roundtable to increase cooperation among patients, providers and payers.

The goal of 80% screening by 2018 goal remains an achievable one. Every person over 50 years of age requires a colonoscopy only every 10 years (if the results are normal). Patients can alternatively undergo a stool Fecal Immunochemical Test (FIT) every year or a stool DNA test (sDNA) every 3 years.

The Louisiana Colorectal Cancer Roundtable and its current statewide iteration, working with providers in the New Orleans area and statewide (including Federal Qualified Health Centers and major health systems) are trying to improve access to colonoscopies. Many patients, especially those with Medicaid, may have issues locating a gastroenterologist willing to perform the test. By working directly together, access should be increased. Once piloted in only in New Orleans, this improved access program should be extended to other parts of the state.

Colorectal cancer remains an avoidable killer. Screening tests should be used with all appropriate candidates (those 50 and above, plus some selected younger people). We must also eliminate the racial disparities that plague colorectal cancer rates. Providers and patients need to pitch in to lower our unacceptable death rates from colorectal cancer, especially among those who are uninsured or receiving Medicaid.

DIABETES TREATMENT: INCREASING COMPLEXITY AND COST

Diabetes rates have increased parallel to the epidemic of obesity in the United States. It now affects over 10% of the adult population, many of whom are unaware they have the disease. Diabetes contributes to strokes, heart disease, neuropathy, renal failure, blindness, peripheral vascular disease and amputations. Morbidity and mortality from diabetes continue to soar, as does the price tag for treatment, reaching $245 billion dollars a year in 2012 (around 20% of the U.S. healthcare budget) and estimated to increase significantly parallel to staggering increases in obesity nationwide.

While Americans seem to have become more health conscious, the ubiquitous presence of processed foods, fast foods, sugary drinks, plus the limited opportunities for physical exercise in many locations, have created the perfect storm for fostering obesity and developing diabetes.

Traditionally, diabetes has been divided into "insulin dependent" and "non-insulin dependent." The former is "juvenile onset diabetes" which is an autoimmune disease that destroys the body's capacity to make insulin. The non-insulin dependent group was traditionally made up of adults, mostly overweight, whose body cannot produce enough insulin for their increased needs (but who often have higher than normal amounts of endogenous insulin) and must take various oral medications.

The distinction between these groups has become blurred in recent times with many "adult onset diabetics" beginning in children and adolescents and many of these patients requiring supplemental insulin, in addition to other medications. The first line of treatment, diet and exercise, associated with significant weight loss, proves unattainable for many diabetic patients.

The dramatic increase in diabetes has been associated with an impressive increase in the number of new non-insulin treatments, many of them with hefty price tags. What follows is a brief review of some of the non-insulin medications, along with their mode of action and administrations. The names here are the scientific rather than brand names. A quick look on Google will help you navigate the many brand names.

1. "Secretogogues," are oral medications that promote insulin release from the pancreas. This group includes glimeprimide, glipizide and glyburide, and the glitinides (Replaginide and Nateglinde.)
2. Biguanides, such as Metformin, decreases liver production of glucose. Rosiglitazone and pioglitazones (Thiozolidinediones) increase the body's sensitivity to its own insulin. They are taken orally.
3. Alpha-Glucosidase Inhibitors are taken orally, but are not absorbed by the digestive track. In the gut, they slow the breakdown of carbohydrates into glucose. This group includes Acarbose and Miglitol, both can cause significant digestive symptoms, including bloating and diarrhea.
4. DPP-4 Inhibitors block the enzyme that degrades GLP-1 (Glucogan-Like Polypeptide), an incretin, a substance that stimulates insulin production in the pancreas. This group includes the oral agents, Sitagliptin and Saxagliptin.
5. GLP-1 Analogs act as synthetic incretins, which enhance insulin secretion, but also delay gastric emptying, reduce liver fat and decrease appetite. Exenatide and Liraglutide, are GLP-1 Analogs, and both require injection.
6. Amylin Analogs (Pranlintide) are injectable, and act by decreasing appetite, slowing gastric emptying and reducing liver output of glucose.
7. Last but least, there are the Sodium-Glucose Linked Transporter (SGLT-2) Inhibitors, which inhibit glucose re-absorption in the kidney by about 90%. The inhibitors are called glifozins and the first available agent was canoglifozin (Invocana). Use of this agent requires a normally functioning kidney and its recent release means that its long-term safety remains to be established.

In addition to these single agents from these various classes, there are hosts of combination medication making use of their complimentary modes of action. Among all diabetic medications, methods of deliver (oral vs. injectable), modes of action, side effects and price vary wildly from one agent to the next. Some older medications (such as metformin) exist in inexpensive generic forms, while the newer agents can cost hundreds of dollars a month.

This amazing diversity of treatment options can be daunting for the physician and confusing and expensive for the patient. Direct advertising, aggressively promoting newer medications, is certainly not the best method by which to choose, either for the patient or the physician. The multiple billion-dollar diabetic drug industry, while responding to our increasing need for diabetic medications, should not make anyone forget the fact that significant weight loss and dietary modifications can greatly help the average diabetic achieve control, often without the need for medications at all!

MELANOMA, NEW HOPE
FOR AN OLD PROBLEM

Although one of the less frequent forms of skin cancer (only 5%), melanomas kill more people than either the much more common basal cell or squamous cellular carcinomas combined. Advanced melanoma cases have only a 15% survival rate and with 120,000 new cases diagnosed each year in the U.S. around 9,000 people will die from their melanoma annually.

While directly proportional to sun exposure (which is cumulative over a lifetime), melanomas can occasionally occur in those with minimal exposure risks. Any skin lesion with irregular borders, very dark coloration (sometimes mottled), and bleeding or rapid growth should be aggressively investigated. As mentioned, mortality from melanoma increases with the stage at diagnosis, which depends on the depth of the lesion and the degree of local, regional or distant spread. The more advance the stage, the worse the prognosis with 85% mortality for Stage IV disease (widely metastatic).

In the past, increasing survival rates has been hampered by the unavailability of effective treatments for widespread, metastatic lesions. Early, superficial and localized melanoma can be removed, with 99% survival rates and long-term cures. Formerly, metastatic disease often involved difficult chemotherapy with lots of side effects and very poor results.

The advent of immunobiological agents, such as *Opdivo®* or nivolumab and *Yervoy®* or ipilimumab, has shown promise as single agents and especially in combination chemotherapy. These agents demonstrated a 22% remission rate in 142 patients at mid-stage of their study, a remarkable finding. That being said, over 50% of the patients reported serious side effects with these medications.

Perhaps the most troubling element, besides side effects, is the significant cost of these agents. Nivolumab (*Opdivo*®) costs around $150,000 for a full year treatment and ipilimumab (*Yervoy*®) costs $120,000 for a four-course treatment. This does not, of course, include the cost of administration of the medications by the hospital or clinic and medical oversight of the treatment.

As with other new, highly sophisticated treatments, the question of cost-benefit ratios arises. On the one hand, prolonging life in individual patients by a few weeks, months or years would seem like a worthy goal. This, of course, would hold true if the treatment was very inexpensive, if cost played no role in the decision-making, or if long-term cure becomes truly feasible

On the other hand, since improvements in life expectancy may be modest and the increased cost often exorbitant, it seems intuitive that there are scant benefits when there are significant expenditures of limited resources for very small gains. Unfortunately, resources are always limited and needs always unlimited, so cost effectively must play a role in the decision making process.

A middle of the road approach proves to be the most prudent, especially when both society and the individual patient share some part in the cost burden. That decision making process, straight forward in theory, still remains fraught with emotions and ethical dilemmas that must be addressed on a case-by-case basis.

So melanoma treatments have made significant progress and, if they continue to improve, the survival rates should increase and the costs should decrease as time goes on. Meanwhile, check your skin frequently and report any unusual, irregular, dark and bleeding lesion to your physician. Avoid excessive sun exposure or tanning. Let the optometrist check for melanoma of the retina during an annual glaucoma check. And, of course, make sure your insurance is comprehensive and up-to-date. Cancer treatments, such as those for melanoma, may impose impressive financial burdens.

OBESITY AND CANCER: A DANGEROUS ASSOCIATION

Obesity carries with it a host of negative consequences. Everyone should be aware that obesity predisposes to diabetes (by increasing the need for insulin from the pancreas). It also contributes to cardiovascular disease either through atherosclerosis or as a by-product of diabetes. What is less well known is that obesity increases the risk for 13 different types of cancers. While the mechanism remains elusive (it probably has to do with the increase in inflammation associated with fat), the fact remains that around 630,000 people in the U.S. are diagnosed each year with one of the 13 obesity-related cancers.

Analyzing the relentless increase in obesity in the U.S. and correlating that with the rise in obesity-related cancers has demonstrated the relationship of cause and effect. There has been a 7% increase in all obesity-related cancers from 2005 to 2014 (parallel to an increase in obesity rates which are now over 30% in the U.S. population and 35% in Louisiana). During the same time period there has been a 13% decrease in cancers not related to obesity. Colon cancer is increased by obesity but has nonetheless dropped by 23% due to more aggressive and accurate detection of early lesions due to increased colonoscopies.

So what are the cancers you are more likely to get if you are obese? And what is the percent increase in risk related to obesity? On the top of the list are esophageal and endometrial (uterine) cancers, increased by 9% and 8% respectively. Cancers of the liver, gallbladder and kidney are all increased by 5%. Stomach and brain cancers (meningiomas) are both increased by 2%, while breast, colorectal, pancreas and multiple myelomas are all increased by 2%. Thyroid and ovarian cancers rise by about 1% in the obese.

Why should this be of great concern? First, around 35% of Louisianans are obese and another third are overweight. Older Americans should be particularly concerned since 60% of all cancers occur in people between 50 and 74 years of age. And women should be especially interested since 55% of these obesity-related cancers are diagnosed in women and only 24% in men. As with many health issues, racial disparities exist with more new cancers diagnosed in Blacks and Whites (proportional to their population) than in other races. Rates of death with both colorectal and breast cancer are also higher in the uninsured and underinsured where Blacks are over-represented.

So what can be done? First and foremost, know your Body Mass Index (BMI) and try to achieve a healthy weight. Inactivity levels exceed 30% in Louisianans versus "only" 20% in other parts of the U.S. Healthy food choices should be stressed, including fresh local produce from farmer's markets and other sources. Screen time should be minimized and family meals encouraged.

From a policy perspective, cities should support "complete streets" where walking, biking and driving can peacefully co-exist. Recreational programs for youth and adults (including seniors) should be encouraged. Safe, affordable housing and decent schools in desirable neighborhoods all contribute to a healthy community. Senior citizens must remain active, both physically and mentally in order to avoid multiple dangers of obesity. Your life might depend on it for a number of reasons, both cardiovascular disease and cancer included.

Have a conversation about your BMI goals and preventative tests (such as colonoscopies and mammograms) with your primary care provider. You can enjoy life more and prolong it by maintaining a healthy weight.

EMERGENCY PREPAREDNESS

LOUISIANA'S DISASTER PREPAREDNESS NETWORK

Although Louisiana has many challenging health-related problems relative to other states, we do have some bright spots in our state rankings. One of these relates to our disaster preparedness activities, which were ranked 3/50 among the states by the American College of Emergency Physicians (ACEP) in 2013.

Our costly previous experiences with a succession of hurricanes and our vulnerable geographic position have conspired to make us very sensitive to and very prepared for disasters. The catastrophe of Hurricane Katrina overwhelmed our state's (and nation's) resources. Since then, much time, effort and money have been devoted to improving our preparedness status.

Louisiana possesses a network of shelters among them the 200,000 square foot permanent State Emergency Shelter at Alexandria (aka "The Megashelter"). Other shelters, managed by the Department of Children and Family Services, are opened on an as-needed basis in other locations and can accommodate almost 30,000 residents who lack their own transportation (or those with "critical transportation needs"), that require sheltering.

State shelters (and their capacities) include: Critical Transportation Needs Shelters (11,500), Medical Special Needs Shelters (1,640), Federal Medical Needs Shelters (1,250), a Sex Offender Shelter (120), an Unaccompanied Minor Shelter (60) and Ambulatory Elderly Shelters (1,828). Point-to-Point Shelters (12,595) are organized by mutual agreement between evacuating parishes and sheltering parishes.

The Critical Transportation Needs Shelters cater to those evacuees "without a ride," while the Medical Special Needs and Federal Medical

Shelters accommodate those with specific medical needs (i.e. brittle diabetes, tube feedings, wound care, oxygen dependence and other complex medical conditions.) All state-sponsored shelters work in collaboration with the Red Cross and other privately sponsored shelters which cater to the general evacuee population with their own private modes of transportation. During an event, the 211 Call Center directs callers to appropriate available shelters.

Despite these efforts, the needs may well exceed the demand in case of a "full coastal evacuation." The difference between needs and resources is called the "needs gap" and there are collaborative agreements with neighboring states to receive evacuees from Louisiana. States participating in these efforts and their capacities (which are subject to change depending on circumstances) include Texas (10,000), Tennessee (3,500), Arkansas (4,000) Georgia (3,000) and possibly Kentucky (3,500), which comes to a total of 24,000 evacuees.

Activation of this vast intra-state and inter-state system requires state and federal emergency declarations. The phases of activation include: (1) preparedness, (2) pre-mobilization, (3) activation, (4) shelter operation and (5) demobilization.

Multiple governmental and non-governmental agencies participate in this mammoth sheltering activity. The Governor's Office of Homeland Security and Emergency Preparedness plays a critical role in coordinating the sheltering response once it is initiated by state and federal emergency declarations. Individual department secretaries (i.e. Department of Children and Family Services and Department of Health and Hospitals) participate in decision-making and implementation, as do the many other participating state agencies and departments (i.e. State Police, Wildlife and Fisheries, National Guard, Department of Transportation and many others.)

Despite this massive governmental initiative, it still remains the responsibility of every individual (and business) to have his or her own disaster plan. Information is available at www.getagameplan.org to assist in developing a personalized response. As with many issues in public health, individual actions, coupled with governmental efforts offer the best opportunity for successful sheltering, for which Louisiana distinguishes itself as a leader among states.

RAIN, RAIN, GO AWAY! SHELTERING DURING THE BATON ROUGE FLOODS

The catastrophic rains of August 2016 precipitated massive flooding across Louisiana, notably around Baton Rouge. It is estimated that 55,000 homes were severally damaged or destroyed and thousands of people were displaced, some to friends and family, others to private or state-run shelters. As with most events, the elderly, especially the sick, pose a particular challenge.

Having lived through many disasters, the citizens of Louisiana demonstrate incredible resilience. That being said, the state and federal government must sometimes step in to fill the gaps. Louisiana has a robust disaster preparedness plan that includes many aspects catering to the elderly ill. Specifically, the Office of Public Health, in collaboration with its sister agencies (The Department of Children and Family Services, the Office of Behavioral Health, the Department of Transportation, Medicaid and other agencies) establish what is known as Medical Special Needs Shelters. Nursing home, group homes and hospitals must have their own point-to-point evacuation plans to similar facilities. But that still leaves vulnerable patient populations that include the elderly ill, many of whom receive home-based services such as home health or home hospice and who cannot go to a general (non-medical) shelter. They necessitate more specialized shelters know as "Medical Special Needs Shelters" (MSNS).

One such Medical Special Needs Shelter was established at the field house on the LSU campus during this current event. Since the Office of Public Health usually mans such shelters with personnel from Region 2 (East Baton Rouge and surrounding parishes) in collaboration with personnel from the Capital Area Human Services District from the same region, the fact that almost a third of these employees were among the many flood victims posed a particular challenge. To meet the manpower needs, other employees from other Office of Public Health regions around the state were enlisted to help open and man the MSNS.

As such, the Medical Special Needs Shelter opened without any significant delays at almost a moment's notice. Beds were installed and the necessary operational needs of logistics, operations, finance and planning were established on site. Within hours, around 60 patients (mostly elderly ill with a variety of conditions from oxygen dependent COPD to dialysis to brittle diabetics) were safely in their cots. The Department of Children and Family Services organized wrap-around services, including food and linens, while certain transportation needs were supplied by the Department of Transportation. A combination of LSU campus police, National Guard and Louisiana State Police supplied security services. The Capital Area Human Services District provided behavioral health and leadership personnel. Other state agencies, such as Medicaid and the Offices of Aging and Citizens with Disabilities contributed as well.

The census in the MSNS rose to about one hundred. By the third day, enough federal assets, including United States Public Health Service Federal Medical Station personnel and two Disaster Medical Assistance Teams (from New Mexico and Alabama), had arrived to make a smooth transition. They assumed medical duties at the MSNS with continued assistance from local Department of Children and Family Services and the Capital Area Human Services District representatives who continued wrap-around services, and behavioral health services and discharge planning respectively.

At the peak, over 20,000 people were also housed in 25 general shelters of all sorts scattered around Baton Rouge. The Red Cross assumed responsibility for these shelters, where only about 1,000 evacuees remained after a week of sheltering. Help from the LSU medical residency programs (and medical volunteers) at the MSNS and at the general shelters proved critical in assuring medical care, which was supplemented by Office of Public Health medical strike teams, formed from OPH personnel from all over the state.

Although a robust sheltering response could not eliminate all the misery inflicted by the flooding of August 2016, it helped to provide food, shelter and medical care to the young and the old alike. The elderly ill had a place to go which catered to their particular needs. The prompt arrival of federal assets, including FEMA, also proved an enormous help. While it took over 17 days for federal help to arrive after Hurricane Katrina and 7 days after Gustav and Ike, it only took 3 days in the catastrophic floods of 2016. What a difference a decade can make!

A TALE OF TWO HURRICANES: HARVEY AND ISAAC

Louisiana suffered the impact of two destructive hurricanes (in the post Katrina era): Hurricane Isaac in August 2012 and Hurricane Harvey in August-September 2017. Both events resulted in the opening of the State Emergency Shelter (aka the "Megashelter") in Alexandria, Louisiana. This paper compares the two events, which prompted the activation of Louisiana's emergency response, and explains the reasons for their successful operation.

As a bit of background, the Megashelter was funded with FEMA dollars in the aftermath of Hurricane Katrina (2005). It was conceived and designed specifically as an evacuation center, one of three such proposed sites: Alexandria, Monroe and Shreveport. Eventually, only the Alexandria facility saw the light of day, being completed in 2010. The 200,000 square foot facility, designed specifically as shelter, is divided into a much larger space for critical transportation needs (CTNS) evacuees and a smaller segment for medical special needs clients (MSNS). The CTNS section can accommodate 2,500 evacuees and the MSNS side can house up to 500 clients or more depending on its configuration. A mezzanine contains a security office, storage, billeting for 88 staff and a catwalk allowing direct observation of all parts of the shelter with the exception of the bathrooms. The ground floor also contains a food "servery," a dry goods distribution center and, adjacent to the MSNS, a small clinical area. A loading dock, generators and other amenities, such as ice machines, warming ovens and industrial refrigerators and freezers are found on the ground floor along with administrative offices.

Although parts of the Megashelter (such as the registration area, dining area and parts of the CTNS) may be used for non-sheltering activities, the building was conceived as a fixed shelter and has served as such during Hurricanes Gustav, Ike, Isaac and Harvey. At a cost of over 27 million dollars and an annual operational cost estimated at around $400,000, the Megashelter represents a major investment by the state of Louisiana in disaster preparedness.

When operational, the Louisiana Department of Children and Family Services (DCFS) serves as the shelter manager, while medical response functions are provided by the Office of Public Health (notably represented by the OPH Region VI or Central Louisiana), the Department of Wildlife and Fisheries, the Department of Agriculture, the Louisiana State Police and National Guard. The Department of Transportation and other agencies of the Louisiana Department of Health (i.e. Behavioral Health, Medicaid, Office of Citizens with Development Disabilities and Office of Aging) all contribute to running the shelter.

Such a complex operation could be fraught with problems, but activities there have been achieved with minimal complications, notably with Hurricanes Isaac (2012) and Harvey (2017). This paper focuses on the medical response (ESF-8), which may serve as a best practice for other entities responsible for handling large-scale evacuations, with or without the luxury of a dedicated shelter.

On Wednesday, August 29, 2012, the rains associated with Hurricane Isaac resulted in extensive, unexpected flooding in St. John's Parish, specifically affecting the city of LaPlace, Louisiana. The resulting evacuations, orchestrated by the State of Louisiana emergency preparedness services, brought 1,597 evacuees to the Megashelter CTNS and another103 to the adjacent MSNS. Many residents who would have qualified for the Medical Special Needs Shelter chose to stay with family members in the Critical Transportation Needs Shelter section.

Since the Office of Public Health, in association with other agencies of the Louisiana Department of Health, is responsible for the medical services (ESF-8), the organization of those services with limited personnel posed a particular challenge. To satisfy the medical needs, OPH worked closely with available EMS contracted services. A first aid station, operating 24 hours a day, was established in the CTNS section. It provided basic services such as blood pressure and glucose checks, albuterol breathing treatments, over the counter medications and simple wound care. During the seven days the Megashelter remained open, 685 patients were seen in the first aid station during the Hurricane Isaac event.

For several hours each day, residents from the Louisiana State University-Health Science Center Family Practice Residency program in Alexandria came in for a "sick call" to see more complicated cases, notably those requiring prescription medications. Of the 685 patients seen in first aid, only 157 patients were referred on for evaluation at the OPH clinic area, where the OPH Regional Medical Director, two OPH APRNs or a family practice resident evaluated them. Since there were no x-ray or lab facilities, the care provided was that of "alternate standards of care" or "field medicine." Nonetheless, only 30 patients were referred out to local ERs and, of those, only 15 were admitted to local hospitals. Thus, of 685 patients seen in the first aid station, only 15 were hospitalized, representing only 2.5% of those treated medically in the shelter and a very manageable burden on our two local hospitals (CHRISTUS St. Frances Cabrini and Rapides Regional Medical Center).

This highly efficient use of resources was duplicated during the Hurricane Harvey (2017) evacuations. On August 31, 2017, after passage of Hurricane Harvey, large swaths of Southeastern Texas received monumental amounts of rain (up to 50 inches total over several days). This resulted in extensive flooding not only in Houston, but also in the towns of Beaumont, Vidor and Orange, Texas, all close to the Louisiana border. Evacuees were first transported to Lake Charles, Louisiana, but were subsequently bused to the Megashelter at Alexandria, Louisiana. Around 2000 evacuees arrived between August 31 and September 1, 2017. Of these 1,840 went to the CTNS and 113 were admitted to the MSNS. Once again, many MSNS eligible evacuees chose to remain with their families in the CTNS sections.

Again, a first aid station, manned 24 hours a day by EMS personnel, was established in the CTNS section of the Megashelter providing over-the-counter medications, blood pressure and serum glucose checks, breathing treatments, simple wound care and other minor services. Residents from the LSU-HSC Family Practice Residency in Alexandria provided more complex care as well as writing prescriptions at the "sick call" several hours each day. Of the 858 evacuees seen at the first aid station, only 214 were referred for an evaluation in the OPH run clinical area adjacent to the MSNS. Of those clients, only 42 were transferred to local ERs. Twenty-two (22) patients were admitted for further care (or 4.5% of those evaluated in the first aid station.)

In addition, the medical residents collaborated with local pharmacies, who sent personnel to the shelter, to provide or renew prescriptions, which were filled and returned to the Megashelter by the pharmacies. This greatly reduced the need for convenience runs (organized by the Department of Transportation) to local pharmacies as had occurred during Hurricane Isaac. Over 900 prescriptions were filled during the Harvey event.

Of particular interest was the problem of narcotic prescriptions. Those were filled only by the OPH Medical Director on a short-term basis and only after consultation with Louisiana's Prescription Monitoring Program (PMP), which has reciprocity with Texas (as well as Arkansas and Mississippi). Around 40 short-term narcotic prescriptions were filled, including hydrocodone (10 prescriptions), clonazepam (6), tramadol (6), alprazolam (5), dihydromorphone (3) and diazepam (2). The reciprocity arrangement between the Louisiana PMP and that of Texas proved an invaluable asset.

The adjacent Ag Center, operated by the Department of Agriculture in collaboration with the Department of Wildlife and Fisheries, housed 208 dogs, 38 cats and 1 bird during the event. All pets were accounted for and returned with their owners who either left the shelter with friends and relatives or were repatriated to Texas after a week in the Megashelter.

While there can always be room for improvement, the organization of medical care with a 24-hour EMS-operated first aid station, supplemented with daily "sick calls," and prescription writing by medical residents, and the use of an OPH clinical area for triage and treatment of more complex cases, proved a highly efficient use of shelter and community resources. Although the OPH clinical area had minimal diagnostic possibilities (an EKG, glucose finger sticks, an oximeter and urine dip sticks) providers (including the medical residents, OPH Medical Director and OPH APRNs) were nonetheless able to provide care, albeit using altered standards of care consistent with field medicine during a disaster.

Sheltering, to be effective, must be a collaborative effort from all of the ESF components. Our experience during Hurricanes Isaac and Harvey demonstrated that cost-effective, high quality services could be delivered even with significant personnel constraints. While all communities do not have the luxury of a fixed shelter facility such as the Megashelter, the model for medical care delivery could be duplicated with limited resources, accompanied by excellent collaboration among all the providers. While we did have some volunteer physician assistance, it would not have been adequate in itself to satisfy the medical needs of the evacuees.

Our experiences with both Hurricanes Isaac (2012) and Harvey (2017) demonstrated that an EMS-driven medical model, with limited mid and upper level providers, can provide for the medical needs of evacuees. There was one birth (in the hospital after referral) and no deaths among the over 3,000 evacuees in these events, a remarkable achievement indeed.

ENVIRONMENTAL ISSUES

HEAT KILLS

Extreme heat kills. In fact, over 7,000 people died from heat-related causes from 1999-2009. Most of these deaths (around 70%) occurred at home and over 90% of those homes lacked functioning air conditioning. Heat kills over 600 people a year, more than those who die from lightning strikes, floods and tornadoes combined. Between 1999 and 2003, 7% of deaths were in children up to 15 years old, 53% were in those between 15 and 64 and 40% were in those 65 and over.

Young children and older people are at higher risk because of an inability to control body heat and a poor response to thirst. Any severe underlying disease, especially diabetes, also increases the risk of heat-related problems.

The signs and symptoms of heat-related disease extend from heat exhaustion to heat stroke. In heat exhaustion, the body is desperately trying to cool down. The person will be sweating profusely and have a rapid, but weak, pulse. They may experience light-headedness, nausea or vomiting, muscle cramps and will feel cool and clammy. Body temperature remains normal until the patient's system fails to keep pace. During heat exhaustion, the patient is usually coherent. Rapid and effective cooling and fluid replacement are imperative to prevent progression to heat stroke.

During heat stroke, the body's capacity to remain cool fails entirely. The core body temperature may soar up to 106 degrees Fahrenheit. The skin turns red, hot and dry and the pulse is rapid and pounding. The person stops sweating and they experience headaches before they become confused and pass out. People in heat stroke will progress to multi-organ failure and die unless they receive medical attention (including aggressive fluid replacement and cooling.) 911 should be called immediately if heat stroke is suspected.

Prevention is, of course, the best medicine. People should avoid extreme physical activity during the heat of the day if at all possible, especially in the South where high humidity prevents effective sweating. Adequate fluids (without alcohol or caffeine), plus light, loose clothing should be encouraged. Air conditioning must be maintained in working order and "cooling centers" can be established in public areas for at-risk individuals.

Since the elderly pay a disproportionate price in mortality, everyone should check on elderly friends, relatives or neighbors. Never leave children (or pets) in an unattended vehicle since temperatures become rapidly fatal. Young infants should not be exposed to extreme heat since they cannot control their body temperature effectively.

In short, enjoy the long, lazy days of summer, but don't let the heat get the best of you. Take care of yourself and remain attentive to those around you. If you must work outdoors, drink plenty of fluids and watch for the signs and symptoms of heat exhaustion. For suspected heat stroke, call 911 immediately. Heat can and does kill. Don't be a victim.

BAD APPLES AND BAD BARRELS, WHY PLACE MATTERS?

Louisiana suffers from a plethora of poor statistics: high obesity, high teenage pregnancy, high infant mortality, high STD (Sexually Transmitted Disease)/HIV rates, high poverty, high incarceration and murder rates. The South, by and large, shares Louisiana's poor outcomes. But even within the region (and the state), the statistics vary greatly from place to place and from group to group.

African-Americans suffer from a disproportionate share of our state's poor health outcomes, much of which can be attributed to poverty and low educational levels. Well-defined pockets of poverty and poor health outcomes remain easily identifiable. While individual choices remain critically important, the environment in which people live has a predictive value on their subsequent behavior and development.

Poor neighborhoods have fewer supermarkets and parks, poorer achieving schools, more crime and correspondingly high rates of STDs, obesity, hypertension, teenage pregnancy, infant mortality, high-school dropouts and crime. The inverse is, of course, true of wealthier neighborhoods creating a disturbing tableau of separate and unequal communities.

The fact remains that, despite remarkable individual examples to the contrary, bad barrels produce bad apples and good barrels produce good apples. While not ignoring the individual apple, the trick for improving results appears to be eliminating bad barrels. Pockets of concentrated poverty (sometimes called "concentrated disadvantage") generate poor outcomes, whether it is a neighborhood, a city, a state or a nation. Professor Zimbardo, in his famous Stanford Prison Experiment, clearly demonstrated that the situation in which people are placed (in his case randomly assigned guards vs. prisoners) could lead to predictable unfavorable results, what he called "The Lucifer Effect."

People who manage to climb out of poverty by personal initiative should be congratulated. But reducing or eliminating "concentrated disadvantage" should be the goal of city planners, policy makers and community activists. "Bad apples" require disproportionate resources, whether it be medical care, education resources, incarceration or other expensive institutionalization. Such resources might be better spent on improving the barrels from which they emerge in order to increase the number of good apples. Place truly matters and both individuals and policy makers can work toward making all the barrels the best ones possible.

While we all can and should make healthy individual decisions, it is much easier when the environment in which we live, work, worship and play is conducive to positive choices. Place really does matter!

Zimbardo, Philip. *The Lucifer Effect: Understanding How Good People Turn Evil*, January 2008.

Dannenberg, AL, H Frumpkin and RJ Jackson. *Making Healthy Places*. Island Press, 2011.

GET THE LEAD OUT!

Lead poisoning can be devastating at any age, but is particularly destructive in very young children due to its effects on the developing brain. The events in Flint, Michigan have only highlighted this long-standing issue of national importance.

Lead is a naturally occurring heavy metal that is also found in older paint (pre-dating 1978), some pipes, folk remedies from various countries (India, China, Thailand, Latin America and elsewhere), soil, some ceramics, environmental dust, water and some traditional cosmetics ("kohl," an eyeliner.) It can also be found in products used in leisure activities such as stained glass window making and hunting (use of lead containing pellets.)

Lead, which accumulates in tissues, can give a variety of symptoms in children including developmental delays, irritability, weight loss, abdominal pain, constipation, fatigue, and hearing loss. Adults can also present with a number of signs and symptoms (notably hypertension, muscle pains, abdominal pains, constipation, headache, mood swings, and declining mental status.) Initial lead exposure in both children and adults may be asymptomatic (no symptoms at all). Physicians must have a high level of suspicion, especially when patients present with a baffling array of seemingly minor and unrelated symptoms.

Treatment of lead poisoning depends on the blood lead levels. At any level, however, it is critical to locate and eliminate the source of exposure. Since lead can be present in many sources in the environment, some detective work may be required. Paint in older housing (prior to 1978) must always be considered, as well as older furniture, toys, pipes, ceramics and traditional remedies and cosmetics. Caregiver education is critical to insure elimination of all sources of lead.

For very elevated blood lead levels (BLL), (i.e. over 45 micrograms/dl), chelation treatments (whether oral or with an EDTA) may be considered, although these must be strictly supervised by a physician. For all elevated levels, regular monitoring of BLL should occur that will document a progressive decrease. Special neurological testing may be required and it is important to remember that developmental surveillance should continue well after diagnosis occurs since the effects of lead poisoning last for years.

Although considerable research and debate has occurred, the scientific consensus is that dietary supplementation with iron, vitamin C and calcium is not required if normal adequate intake is assured and previous deficiencies do not exist. For environmental sources, simple measures like hand washing, wet mopping floors, leaving shoes at the door, avoiding direct soil content, and using cold tap water for drinking and cooking can help in reducing exposure. Any lead related to hobbies (stained glass, use of lead pellets for hunting, furniture restoration, car batteries, and others) should be identified and eliminated. To reassure the public, water systems in Louisiana are regularly tested by the Department of Health, Office of Public Health, and elevated levels are aggressively addressed.

Fortunately, pediatricians screen for blood lead levels (BLL) during routine well-child exams, although there are some practitioner variations in when and how often this occurs. Blood lead surveillance is tracked nationally since at least 1997 and the results have shown a dramatic reduction in the percentage of children with confirmed elevated BLL above 10 micrograms/deciliter (from 7.61% in1997 to 0.53% in 2014). This has also been the case for Louisiana, where the percent of children tested with elevated BLL fell from 2.38% (1998) to 0.67% (2014) out of over 375,000 infants and children tested. There is some discussion recently about reducing the acceptable thresholds even lower.

Despite these dramatic decreases from previous decades, we still need to have broad public awareness of this problem, which still remains an avoidable threat to infants and adults. It's time for us all to get the lead out!

NOISE POLLUTION

The problem posed by noisy vehicles has existed throughout history. Chariots, clattering over paving stones, were so disruptive to sleep that they were limited to daytime use in ancient Rome. In Medieval Europe, the cobblestones were covered with straw to reduce noise, while dirt was used over paving stones in colonial Philadelphia. Noise is a ubiquitous and disruptive problem recognized by 30% of Americans in the 2000 census, 40% of whom were considering a change in address to alleviate noise irritation.

After passage of the Noise Protection Agency in 1972, the U.S. Environmental Protection Agency founded the Office of Noise Abatement and Control, which was subsequently closed in 1982. There was a proliferation of local noise ordinances as well, which may or may not be effective in addressing the noise problem.

Why is this important? Perhaps foremost, "Domestic Tranquility" is guaranteed in the U.S. Constitution. This does not prevent over 100 million Americans from being exposed daily to unsafe levels of noise. Such exposure leads to a number of unpleasant or dangerous effects. The first is hearing loss, precipitated by exposure to noise levels at or exceeding 85 decibels (dB). Heavy truck traffic creates around 90 dB, while firecrackers or a subway train generate 100 dB, and a rock concert or jet traffic cause about from 110-120 dB. A monster truck generates around 110 dB, while a monster truck event can produce over 130 dB, clearly dangerous to spectators and participants. The risk of permanent hearing loss is directly proportional to the cumulative duration of the exposure to noise, the longer, the worse the loss.

Other negative effects of loud noise include interference with normal conversations, sleep disturbance and even cardiovascular problems such as increased heart rate and blood pressure, both of which increase the risk of heart disease. Long-standing and repetitive noise pollution also results in mental health issues such as anxiety, depression and irritability, negative social behavior and annoyance reactions, all associated with a decrease in quality of life and job performance. Each of the above negative effects is more acute in the very young and very old, both of whom lack coping mechanisms.

If loud, repetitive noises are so destructive, why are they allowed? First, many local noise ordinances can be vague, non-specific and poorly enforced, if at all. Many local law enforcement agencies have neither the willingness nor the time to worry about such an "unimportant" problem. Given the host of negative effects, however, this issue should be given the upmost priority.

Currently, the Rapides Parish Police Jury, Louisiana, Code of Ordinances, Article II. Noise, addressed this problem since July 10, 1990. It states: *"Unnecessary noise prohibited. It shall be unlawful for any person to make, continue or cause to be made or continued any loud, unnecessary or unusual noise or any noise which either annoys, disturbs, injures or endangers the comfort, repose, health, peace or safety of others within the parish."* Unfortunately, there are no specific references to the agreed upon danger level of 85 dB or higher. The time restriction for noise control appears to be only limited between 11:00 p.m. and 7:00 a.m., a period that would not cover the sleeping times of many citizens, especially the elderly and very young.

Noise pollution clearly represents a danger to health and a violation of our Constitutional right to "Domestic Tranquility." There is ample opportunity to add specificity (notably decibel levels over 85 or surely 100) and more stringent time restrictions to the current parish legislation. We all deserve some peace and quiet for our mental and physical health, especially our senior citizens.

Goines, L, L. Hagler, (2007) Noise Pollution: A Modern Plague. Southern Medical Journal. 100(3) :287-294.

PUBLIC HEALTH AND THE
BUILT ENVIRONMENT

The relationship between the "built environment" and health outcomes has become a hot topic. Research, some of which comes from the Pennington Biomedical Research Center in Baton Rouge, has confirmed that the best approach to improving health involves a dual approach: (1) Education directed toward behavior modification and (2) Environmental policies that promote enhancement of a healthy built environment.

What does this mean? First, everyone has been bombarded with public service announcements for smoking cessation, increased activity, safe sleep, breastfeeding and obesity, which are directed at changing individual choices. Second, these initiatives directed toward individual behavior, however, must be associated with environmental changes, often precipitated by policy change. Examples would be smoke-free areas, promotion of breastfeeding, parks and other recreational amenities.

Asking people to increase their activity makes no sense if there are no places to exercise and no incentives to do so. It has been demonstrated that people who live in proximity to parks are more likely to engage in physical activity. Cities with adequate green spaces, bike trails, and walking trails, promote health in a more direct way than simply encouraging people to get up and move. That being said, those individuals who live in low-income, high crime neighborhoods are less likely to benefit from the proximity of green spaces than those in high-income, low-crime areas. From a purely policy prospective, initiatives such as reducing health insurance premiums for those with normal weights and who do not smoke, and who engage in regular health check-ups would be examples.

Progressive communities have seized on research findings and incorporate "public health in all policies." Baton Rouge has the "Mayor's Health City Initiative," which promotes healthy lifestyles, accessible quality clinical care and research into a triple faceted program. Advisory boards head up the three parts of this initiative, which targets priorities as diverse as obesity, HIV/AIDS, mental health access and overutilization of emergencies rooms. Given Louisiana's poor health outcomes, all such projects can only improve our standings compared with other states.

With respect to the "obesity priority," Baton Rouge's response has been, among other things, development of a mobile farmer's market, improvement of school equipment and activity programs, promotion of the 5-2-1-0-10 program (5 servings of fruits and vegetables, 2 hours or less of screen time per day, 1 hour of exercise a day, 0 sweet drinks, and 10 hours of sleep), encouragement of farm to school fruit and vegetable use and the "Baton Rouge on the Geaux" van. They have also completed an ambitious walking trail passing by the Mall of Louisiana and several of the major medical facilities.

This multifaceted program hopes to reduce obesity, especially among the 30% of Baton Rouge children who are already affected. No single group and no single approach can be successful when the problem itself has so many diverse origins. Alexandria, in collaboration with the Rapides Foundation and other entities, has embarked in similar initiatives to tackle similar health issues in our regional community and should be supported whenever possible. Alexandria's annual recreation summit represents another positive step. The long-term health of our citizens is at stake.

SUMMERTIME DANGERS: WATER RELATED ILLNESSES

Summer fun often includes water and that can be in public pools, water parks, ponds, rivers or bayous. Fresh water fun, however, does have its share of potential hazards beyond the risk of drowning. The list of potential infectious illnesses that can come from fresh water exposure includes cryptosporidia, giardia, shigella, norovirus, E. Coli and the much publicized, albeit rare, Naegleria fowleri.

Cryptosporidia is a parasitic infection, transmitted by the fecal-oral route and is the leading cause of pool-related outbreaks of diarrhea. The oocysts of cryptosporidia are highly resistant to chemicals and can survive in treated water. "Crypto" causes acute watery diarrhea and abdominal cramping which can lead to dehydration or even death in immunocompromised hosts.

Giardia, a protozoan or one-celled organism, also includes cysts and trophozoites as part of its life cycle, both of which can be infectious. While infected individuals may be asymptomatic, Giardiasis can cause acute or chronic diarrhea, especially in children. It is most common in untreated bodies of water such as lakes, ponds and streams (or bayous) where it can be transmitted by fecal contamination by either humans or animals (beavers.) While Giardia can be treated with metronidazole (Flagyl®), it is often self-limiting (resolves by itself.)

Shighella, a bacterial disease, also causes an acute self-limiting diarrhea of variable intensity. Transmission can occur through contaminated water or by fecal-oral transmission within a household, where up to 40% of household members may be infected. Antibiotics may be useful, depending on the sensitivity of the organism.

Norovirus, the cruise ship nemesis, is a highly contagious viral infection. Outbreaks of norovirus can sweep through nursing homes and cruise ships alike. And, as with most viral diseases, treatment remains symptomatic during the week or so of acute diarrhea. Adequate cleaning of any infected facility (or cruise ship) remains the mainstay of preventing re-infections.

E. Coli 0157-H7 is one of the main serotypes of E. Coli and causes 90% of the cases of Hemolytic Uremic Syndrome (HUS), a very serious complication of infection with this organism. HUS occurs in less than 8% of E. Coli 0157-H7 infections, but can be life-threatening since it causes destruction of red blood cells and associated renal failure. Most causes of E. Coli 0157-H7 occur with infected food, but water contaminated either with human or cattle feces can also be a source.

Last but not least, Naegleria fowleri, an amoeba (or amoeba-flagellate, a single-celled free-living organism), can also be found in untreated or inadequately treated water alike. Several highly publicized cases in Louisiana resulted in death by meningoencephalitis. Public health changes subsequently occurred, resulting in more stringent chlorination standards. Naegleria fowleri also occurs naturally in fresh water lakes and bayous. Getting water, especially untreated, up the nose should be avoided since the bony separation between the roof of the nasal cavity and the brain is razor thin and perforated by tiny holes (cribriform plate), easily penetrated by an amoeba.

While most of these infectious agents cause diarrhea (with the exception of Naegleria fowleri), the other symptoms they cause resemble one another. Differentiating one from another, while often unnecessary, generally requires a stool sample (or, as Dr. Raoult Ratard, Director of the Louisiana Epidemiology and Infectious Diseases program puts it, "The proof is in the poop"). Not drinking untreated fresh water, hand washing and not allowing soiled diapers in public pools go a long way to reducing outbreaks. If symptoms of diarrhea develop, be sure to remain hydrated since dehydration poses the most common risk, especially to infants and the elderly.

Speaking of children and water, besides the above-mentioned infections, drowning remains the greatest danger. As a state, Louisiana has the 3rd highest rates of childhood drownings in the U.S. For children aged

1-4 years old, drowning is the leading cause of unintentional injury in our state. Most of the drownings were in pools, tubs or spas (47%), while only 26% occurred in lakes, rivers, ponds, creeks or bayous. Lack of supervision was a contributing risk factor in 42% of drowning deaths. While around twelve children die each year from drowning in Louisiana, another 28 young children (1-4 years old) are hospitalized. A proportionately higher percentage of African-American children die from drowning than Whites.

You can still have fun in the water this summer, but remember the hidden dangers that may be lurking from infections. And, of course, children always require strict supervision and should be taught to swim as early as possible.

GO FURTHER WITH FOOD

March happens to be National Nutrition Month and the theme this year was "Go Further with Food." There is a double meaning here, since it hopes to address the use of better food choices as fuel, but also reduction of our massive amounts of food wastage.

Food wastage in the U.S. reaches staggering proportions. It is estimated that 60 million tons of food (or 50% of all produce, worth about $160 billion) is discarded every year. This amounts to a third of all food, most of it ending up in landfills where it represents the largest component. An American family of four throws away over $1,500 of produce annually. Worldwide, the waste is also about a third of all food, sometimes for different reasons such as harvesting and transport issues, but still at a cost of $3 trillion/year.

Why have we become such a wasteful society? There are various reasons, but one driver is the low cost of food in the U.S. as compared with other countries, some of which is related to generous agricultural subsidies. There is also consumer demand, which favors perfect looking produce and rejects anything that might be bruised, wilted or discolored, regardless of how the item will be prepared. Supermarkets recognize this consumer demand for perfection and pre-emptively throw away anything that looks deformed or blemished in any way.

Farmers also pre-emptively eliminate produce that lacks consumer appeal in response to unrelenting consumer demands for the perfect looking product. Our Facebook photo culture aggravates the problem by compelling retailers and restaurants to make picture perfect dishes or risk the ire of hypersensitive consumers and foodies.

A move toward acceptance of local crops, diversity of products, and a shift in esthetics can all help reduce waste. On a personal level, the consumer can take a few useful steps: (1) Take an inventory of food in your home before going to buy more, (2) Buy only limited quantities of food that correspond to what can be eaten or frozen for a few days only, (3) Prepare and serve reasonable portions that contain all food groups, but not in excessive quantities, (4) Buy limited quantities (not the "economy" pack) rather than being obliged to discard what you cannot reasonably consume, (5) Exercise adequately to burn off calories rather than accumulate them as fat, (6) Recycle through composting, (7) Donate unwanted food to food pantries and (8) Learn about the meaning of food labeling (i.e. "Use by," "best by" and "sell by").

In Europe, the refrigerators are tiny by American standards. European housewives will often shop daily, not weekly, at a market or grocery store within walking distance. Produce in a market is usually locally grown and may not be picture perfect. Prices at such markets, however, are usually lower than in a supermarket and thus a sound consumer choice, not a privilege of the wealthy. France and Germany both oblige supermarkets to compost or donate unsold or expiring food.

Louisiana prides itself on its rich and varied food culture. It does not have to be wasteful or unhealthy since an abundance of local products remain available. Eat a healthy breakfast and remain active throughout the day. Celebrate National Nutrition Month (and all year around) by eating right, exercising and reducing waste following the instructions above. If you have specific issues and concerns, do not hesitate to consult a nutritionist who will be happy to explain food choices and their consequences. *Bon appetit*!

GERIATRICS

A HAPPY AND HEALTHY NEW YEAR FOR CENLA'S SENIORS

The beginning of each year marks the time for those inevitable New Year's resolutions. Every year, many of them should be directed toward your health. Here are a few that you might consider:

1. Try and achieve your healthy body mass index (or at least lose 10% of your body weight) if you are either obese or just overweight. Over 60% of our regional population falls in this group, which often suffers from diabetes and all of its terrible complications. Excess weight did not come overnight and it will not leave overnight. There are no quick fixes to obesity, so just reduce your calorie intake (less food) and increase your exercise (if only by 20 minutes of walking every day.) Rigorous fad dieting and expensive supplements are not helpful and almost invariably fail in the long run.

2. Get vaccinated for all of the adult vaccinations. That should include your annual flu shot, which you should take early (in October), but can take as late as March. The strain of flu changes from year to year (due to antigenic shifts and drifts), so you need to take the new shot every year. If you have not done so already, get your pneumonia shot (Prevnar-13® and Pneumovax®) if you are 65 or older. Pneumonia is still the number one killer of the elderly even though people live much longer now than they did a century ago. If you have grandchildren or great-grandchildren, don't forget your TdaP (tetanus, diphtheria, and pertussis). Whooping cough (caused by pertussis) can be carried by adults and given to young

infants, who can then get seriously ill or die. Before you hold that newborn, get the TdaP! Last, but not least, the herpes zoster vaccination (Shingrix® or the older Zostavax®) can save you from the misery of shingles, or at least make it less severe. Although the vaccine is costly, it is worth the money if you can escape from the torment of shingles and post-herpetic neuralgia.

3. Go to your doctor and have him or her check all of your medications. Seniors take a disproportionate amount of medications, some necessary, some not. Make sure everything you take is safe, effective and not interacting with something else you may be taking. That being said, don't self-medicate and that includes pain medications, alcohol and illicit drugs. Seniors are particularly susceptible to all sorts of drugs, both legal and illegal. An unnecessary fall, induced by medications or alcohol, could be the ticket to the hospital with an unwanted fractured hip.

4. Don't forget your end-of-life decisions and documentation. If you have not already done so, you need to create or review your will, designate a power of attorney, formulate a living will, and have frank discussions with family members about your wishes. No one really wants to have these discussions, but it is far better to have them when you can participate than when you may be unable to do so.

5. Make your home elder-safe. Remove slippery throw rugs, install grip bars in the bathrooms, remove unnecessary cords, insure adequate lighting, and make sure you know who to contact and how in case of an emergency. Don't forget the smoke alarm and carbon monoxide alarms either. If your neighborhood has safety issues, an alarm system should be considered. If you have guns, make sure they are locked up so they do not become a safety hazard for you or your family. Seniors commit suicide with their own gun far more often than they foil a would-be intruder. And as with younger populations, don't text and drive either.

6. Don't neglect your mental health. Depression is not a normal part of aging. Remaining mentally and physically active improves personal satisfaction and longevity. If you are depressed, be sure to seek medical help. Safe and effective medications exist, although

their doses may have to be adjusted for your age. Socialize and surround yourself by positive individuals, who care about you and your welfare. Make sure friends and family visit regularly to check on you. Home health services can also be wonderful, when medically indicated.

In short, set your sights for a healthy and happy New Year. Aging is not for the faint hearted, since it brings with it a host of challenges. Yet it can also be one of the happiest times of life. As the poet Robert Browning wrote, "Grow old along with me! The best is yet to be, the last of life for which the first was made."

ARTHRITIS: A COSTLY PROBLEM

Arthritis is a ubiquitous problem, with one American in four (or 54 million) suffers from some form of arthritis. This includes osteoarthritis (the most common), but also includes gout, lupus, fibromyalgia, rheumatoid arthritis or some other less common variants. Any form of arthritis has a negative impact on activity and around 24 million adults report a limitation in their activities attributed to their arthritis. Since our population is also aging rapidly, the problem will only increase from our current 54 million affected adults in 2015 to over 78 million by 2040, a 30% increase.

Although we associate arthritis with the elderly, over half of arthritis sufferers are between 18 and 64 years old (working age) the economic implications are staggering. It is estimated that arthritis costs over $81 billion a year in direct medical costs and probably at least as much in indirect costs. There has been a 20% increase in adults reporting limitations of their activities (24 million) unrelated to aging over the last several years.

Adults with arthritis are twice as likely to report falls and are more likely to be unemployed. Comorbidities with arthritis include heart disease (49%), diabetes (47%) and obesity (31%), all of which are complicated by the accompanying arthritis. Chronic arthritis has also disproportionately contributed to the opioid crisis, despite the fact that opioids are rarely indicated for chronic pain of any kind, especially in the elderly.

Besides decreasing mobility, one third of arthritis sufferers report depression, about the same percentage as have problems bending, stooping or kneeling. Over 20% of arthritis sufferers cannot walk three blocks or more. And since African-Americans and Hispanics are more likely to be obese, their comorbidity associated with weight-related arthritis is correspondingly higher than Whites. Women suffer more arthritis than men, and represent about 60% of all sufferers. In short, many individuals of both sexes, all races and all age groups suffer from arthritis.

So what can be done? First, arthritis is not inevitable or necessarily debilitating. Regular physical activity such as walking, swimming, biking, or even dancing, can be helpful. Second, providers should encourage reasonable physical activities for both delaying arthritis and achieving weight reduction. Cooperation among healthcare providers, public health, parks and recreations departments and city planners is crucial. Third, community-based organizations should address the problem of arthritis before the consequences become more expensive and debilitating. Fourth, opioids should be avoided for arthritis, as well as for most other chronic conditions in order to reduce the ravages of long-term drug addiction.

Together we can find solutions for this vexing and expensive problem.

COME GROW OLD WITH ME, THE BEST IS YET TO BE, OR IS IT?

Despite Robert Browning's comforting quote ("Come grow old with me, the best is yet to be,") growing old is not for the timorous. Ready or not, however, as a society we will be confronted by a tidal wave of seniors over the next decades. On the crest of this tidal wave are, of course, the notorious baby boomers. By 2030, 20% of the population will be over 65. Over the next twenty years, the number of Americans 65 and older will double from around 36 million to over 72 million. This number will reach a staggering 89 million by 2050.

Since seniors add their accumulated wit, wisdom and wealth to society, it should be a win-win for everyone. Alas, seniors also bring with them the liability of increased illness and the corresponding increased costs of medical care. Around 80% of seniors have at least one chronic disease, while 66% have at least two chronic conditions and 40% suffer from three or more chronic diseases. Just as seniors leave the work force, they add medical costs to the society. Medicare expenditures reached $536 billion in 2012 and rose to $592 billion by 2013 and will reach an astonishing $1.1 trillion by 2023. As a point of comparison, all combined medical expenditures in the U.S. in 2014 were "only" $3 trillion, or about 18% of the U.S. Gross Domestic Product (GDP).

While the increase in per capita Medicare spending has slowed to 0.4% in 2012 (down from 3.6% in 2011), the sheer number of beneficiaries risks breaking the national bank. Overuse, especially of new, hugely expensive medications and technologies, contribute to increased costs. While "managed care," (such as in Medicare Advantage), and certain elements of the Affordable Care Act (such as Accountable Care Organizations and

Patient Homes) have helped to blunt the curb of rising costs, the tsunami of spending is still ready to submerge us all. Abolition of elements of Obamacare may further exacerbate the problem by allowing younger, healthier individual to forgo medical insurance altogether.

Of special interest is long-term care, an inevitable significant future expenditure. Over 70% of American seniors will need long-term services and supports, for which Medicaid is the primary payer (40% of the $357 billion). The vast majority (87%) of those requiring care will rely on unpaid family members, an additional hidden burden to society. While most American seniors recognize their probable need for long-term care, a mere 35% have set aside money for that purpose, leaving the burden for relatives or for society at large to shoulder. Those who assume that Medicare will take care of them ignore the fact that Medicare does not provide long-term care coverage.

More seniors, increased longevity, long-term care costs, increased morbidity and the rising costs for medications and technology all conspire to form a perfect, catastrophic storm. There are some suggested solutions to this impending crisis, however, which include: (1) an emphasis on preventive medicine and wellness, (2) using care coordinators to manage chronic conditions, (3) decreasing unnecessary procedures and tests, (4) restricting the use of the latest and invariably more expensive medications, (5) reducing administrative costs, (6) managing terminal illnesses in a more sensible manner (7) and achieving meaningful tort reforms (however unlikely) to our contingency fee driven malpractice crisis.

The devil, of course, lies in the details. Everyone demands the latest, best technology and the newest, most expensive medications, encouraged by an avalanche of direct to consumer advertising. We also demand perfect outcomes and the right to sue at "no cost" if perfection is not achieved. And why not? We have contributed to Medicare and now we have the right to expect the best and most expensive treatments. But do we?

The baby boomers, the crest of the tidal wave, have always distinguished themselves by a streak of self-indulgence and self-centeredness. Rightfully called the "me" generation, baby boomers should accept the fact that illness and death are a part of life. And while we do not necessarily need to "go quietly into that night," we must accept the responsibility of leaving a sustainable society to our children and grandchildren. When those same loved ones and progeny scream to "do everything" to the doctors in the ER or ICU, we need to have the common sense and courage to respond that "everything" may not be the best for any of us. That decision needs to be codified in a living will that keeps conflict away from the bedside.

DIVORCE AMONG THE ELDERLY, THE GRAY DIVORCE REVOLUTION

Although perhaps not a major public health issue, divorce among the elderly is on the rise. In the 1960's, only 2.8% of Americans 50 and older were divorced. This figure jumped to 11.8% by 2000, and to 15.4% by 2011. This means that currently, more Americans 50 or older are divorced than widowed (13.5%). Coupled with an increase in the elderly population, these divorce numbers are estimated to increase by 25% over the next two decades.

Once again, the baby boomers have led the pack. The chances of divorce increase with second and third marriages and these have become increasingly common among boomers. One in four divorces (25%) are now in older Americans, up from one in ten in 1990. Divorces among those 65 and older have jumped from 5% in 1990 to 7.4% in 2002.

So what precipitates divorce among the elderly? An empty nest tops the list. Those who have devoted their lives to their children, and then find themselves face-to-face when their children are gone, face particular challenges. Midlife crises play another role, with individuals suffering from a sense of alienation, while seeking the excitement and stimulation of a new, often younger partner. Wives, who are the most likely to initiate a divorce, generally cite infidelity and emotional abuse as triggers, while men cite loss of love and incompatibility.

Sadly, illness also precipitates a divorce by inflicting unsustainable demands on one of the partners. The emotional cost is compounded by the financial burden of long-term care or expensive medical treatments. Divorce sometimes becomes the only way to maintain at least one financially healthy partner while the other must rely on Medicaid. A similar phenomena of untoward stress ending in divorce can occur with the emotional burden of a lost child, especially when untreated or unrecognized depression occurs in one or both of the parents.

Experts advise to be on the lookout for warning signs of a deteriorating couple such as (1) an emotional disconnect between one person seeking more quality time together and the other being too tired or distracted, (2) withdrawal into excessive work, all-consuming hobbies, unreasonable exercise programs or intense outside separate friendships, (3) decline in intimacy and loss of romance, (4) and excessive laptop or I-phone time with virtual friends.

While a subsequent healthy relationship is established in 75 to 80% of divorced elderly, especially if they are financial well-off and well-educated, divorce can be devastating. Older women may not have their own pensions, which husbands refuse to share, and these women can lack the skills and stamina for the job market. This is especially true of Hispanic and African-American women. Adult children of divorced elderly can also aggravate the situation by resenting one or the other of their parents, increasing their emotional distress.

Despite an anticipated 25% increase in elderly divorce in the coming decades, the good news remains that the longer a couple has been married, the more likely the marriage is to survive. Education and wealth increase your chances of marital survival, as does a constant effort to cultivate the love life of the couple over the years. Around two thirds of all "gray" divorces can be prevented with counseling and education. So spend some quality time with your spouse! We can still have said "'til death do us part" and have meant it, even though we are living longer than ever.

EXERCISE AND THE ELDERLY

Once you hit 50, there is a temptation to reduce or eliminate exercise. There are a number of common excuses including: the inevitability of aging, the need to save one's strength, the risk of falls, or the idea that you are too old to start exercising and nothing good will come of it. Each excuse is wrong and the advantages of regular exercise are extraordinary.

First, exercise helps you maintain your normal body weight. With age, many people pack on unnecessary pounds that only increase their risk for diabetes, heart disease, osteoporosis, colon cancer and even Alzheimer's disease. Second, exercise increases muscle strength and endurance, both of which decrease the risk for falls and the possibility of a hip fracture. Third, people who exercise retain a better mental outlook, with higher self-esteem, better sleeping habits and enhanced intellectual abilities.

The recommended goal for exercise is at least 150 minutes of aerobic activity during the week. Hopefully, this can be increased to 300 minutes of exercise a week, with intense physical activity occurring in 10-minute bouts. Whatever the level of exercise you attain, it should be a mixture of the four goals of any program: (1) cardio-endurance, (2) strength and power, (3) flexibility and (4) balance. Each of these goals uses rhythmic motions, repetitive motions, full range motions, and stability exercises respectively, or some combination of all four.

Since older individuals may have pre-existing health issues, it is always prudent to talk to your primary care physician before embarking on an aggressive exercise program. That being said, even being wheelchair bound does not prevent a modified exercise regimen that will be equally beneficial. Whatever the immediate or long-term health goals, it is best to choose activities you enjoy. If you choose dancing, hiking, gardening, yoga, Tai Chi or martial arts, you are more likely to stick with a program containing activities you like.

Once you have decided to embark on an exercise program, start slowly and build up gradually. And then stick with it at least a month or more until it becomes part of your daily routine. Don't neglect the social aspect of exercise either. When you move with others, you engage in "social sweat," creating muscle mass and friendships at the same time. You do not, however, need special equipment, individual trainers, or an expensive gym membership. Make even day-to-day activities such as house cleaning, shopping, gardening or caring for grandchildren opportunities to push, pull, stretch, climb and balance.

If any of your activities cause shortness of breath, dizziness, chest pain, ankle swelling or persistent joint or muscle pains, stop what you are doing and consult your physician. Senior citizens can and should exercise, but prudence and common sense must always prevail.

www.helpguide.org/life/senior_fitness_sports.htm

FLU VACCINE AND THE ELDERLY: IT'S A MUST!

Influenza (or "the flu") usually occurs as a seasonal illness between October and April each year. Occasionally, a "pandemic" takes place that continues beyond the usual season, such as occurred with H1N1 (the swine flu). Either way, flu kills. Annual deaths vary from 3,000 to 50,000 a year, depending on the severity of the stains. The most vulnerable populations (with some exceptions) are young children and people over 65 years of age.

The elderly are particularly prone to complications of the flu because of the decreased immunity that occurs with age and the frequency of other co-morbid conditions, notably diabetes, kidney disease and chronic obstructive lung disease (COPD.) While flu vaccination rates are better among older Americans (around 66%) than younger adults (35% for those from 20-64), they are far from the Healthy People 2020 goal of 90%.

What havoc does the flu cause each year? Besides the very real risk of death (around 5,500 seniors over 65 each year on average), over 2.3 million senior citizens got the flu in the 2012-2013 season, 1.3 million sought medical attention and over 200,000 were hospitalized. The 2017-2018 proved to be equally bad, if not worse, with an aggressive H3N2 flu strain, only partially covered by the flu vaccine for that season.

So does the shot do any good? Again, much like the severity of the flu itself, the vaccine effectiveness may vary from year to year, although it is still very useful. In the 2011-2012 season, the vaccine reduced flu-related hospitalizations by 60 to 77%, with significant impacts among diabetics and those with COPD of any age. During the 2012-2013 flu season, vaccinations prevented an estimated 44,000 hospitalizations, 270,000 medical visits, and prevented nearly 500,000 cases in seniors. Flu vaccination prevents the death of one older person for every 4,000 seniors vaccinated, certainly worth the time and effort. Even when protection runs as low as 10 to 30%, flu vaccination still blunts the severity of the illness and may well mean the difference between life and death in the profoundly ill.

The composition of the vaccine varies from year to year based on prevailing strains of the Influenza A. The CDC now recommends that everyone older than 6 months (and surely those over 65) get vaccinated every year. Those at especially high risk of flu complications include everyone over 65, those with diabetes, heart disease, asthma, HIV, kidney disease and COPD. Only those allergic to the flu vaccine itself or who have suffered from Guillian-Barré Syndrome (a rare neurological disorder) should refrain from getting vaccinated. Once administered, the vaccine takes a couple of weeks to stimulate immunity. Even so, being recently vaccinated with some immunity is better than not being vaccinated at all.

Despite rumors to the contrary, you cannot "get the flu" from the inactivated influenza vaccine. You can, however, get some minor redness and swelling at the site of injection, or some headache and muscle aches lasting a couple of days at most. Remember that the flu spreads from person to person with coughing and sneezing, or ingestion of infected droplets picked up in the environment where it may live up to 24 hours. Cough into your sleeve or use a tissue, wash your hands regularly, and stay at home until you get better in order to reduce the risk of contagion. Exercise "social distancing" if you are ill, remaining at a distance from everyone as much as possible. Your flu infection doesn't need to be shared with everyone.

HEARING LOSS: A COMMON AND PREVENTABLE PROBLEM

Around 40 million U.S. adults suffer from hearing loss attributed to exposure to noise. Hearing loss is common and occurs twice as often as diabetes or cancer. Noise exposure, the usual culprit, may be on the job or at home. Either way, the louder or longer the exposure, the greater the damage.

Those at highest risk include those exposed to more than 85 decibels (noise from a leaf blower) for more than 8 hours a day and males over 40 years of age. Although most people blame a noisy work environment for damage to hearing, over half of people with hearing loss are not working in a noisy environment. And a fifth of people with hearing loss never worked in a noisy environment. Hearing loss, independent of ambient noise exposure, increases with age, with only 7% suffering hearing loss among those 20 to 30 years old and rising steeply to 68% in the 60 to 69 age group.

While some with hearing loss may never have worked in a noisy environment, continual loud noise exposure, whatever the source, not only damages hearing, but also contributes to stress, anxiety, hypertension, heart disease, depression and may even contribute to dementia. Some risk factors for hearing loss include a history of prolonged noise exposure (whether at work, home or recreationally), male sex and being 40 years of age or older. Hearing loss can be insidious, so 25% of those who have measurable loss are unaware of any changes at all.

The cost of hearing loss treatment was estimated at $8 billion in 2002 and projected to rise to $51 million by 2030. Those with hearing loss incur 33% higher health care costs than those without it. Despite the staggering cumulative costs, over 70 % of those exposed to loud noises wear no ear protection. When people do begin to lose their hearing, about 45% will not have consulted with a doctor or audiologist and thus remain untreated.

Health care providers need to be aware of the problem of hearing loss and recognize those at greatest risk. Patients should be warned to avoid noisy environments, wear ear protection and seek medical evaluations if they notice any changes. Because of the frequency of hearing loss, those over 60 should consider being tested, at least once, by an audiologist. City planners, employers and policy makers need to be aware of the noise created in the city and in the workplace. There needs to be a willingness to collaboratively address the problem at work, at home and in the built environment.

Hearing loss is a costly tragedy, especially when it is preventable. It is important to reduce risk factors when possible and encourage people to overcome their reticence to be evaluated so effective treatments, if any, can be initiated.

WHAT GRANDPARENTS AND PARENTS NEED TO KNOW ABOUT INFANT DEATHS IN LOUISIANA

Although it may seems like a topic for young parents, grandparents often end up raising their grandchildren, or at least become actively involved with assisting the parents. As such, they need to know the dreadful statistics about infant deaths in Louisiana. Many factors contribute to fetal and infant deaths. As with most unfavorable health outcomes, three factors always contribute: poverty, low educational level and low social status (the SES or "socioeconomic factors.") In Louisiana, as in other states, these factors become inextricably tied with race, either African-American or Hispanic, resulting in disparities in health outcomes so omnipresent in Southern states.

The fact remains that more infants die in Louisiana than in almost any other state. For 2016, Louisiana ranked 48/50 for its infant mortality (8.1/1,000 live births). This dropped slightly in 2017 to 7.6/1,000 live births, still much higher than the national average of 5.9/1,000 live births. The infant mortality among African-Americans (11.7/1,000 live births) was much higher than that for Whites (5.8/1,000). More babies died when the mothers were 15-19 (10.9/1,000) and was lowest among mothers 25-29 (6.09/1,000). Such grim statistics, always worse for those with low socio-economic status (where Blacks are overly represented), are even unequally distributed throughout Louisiana. The Central and Northern Mississippi River parishes suffer worse outcomes, including those for low birth weights (directly correlated with infant mortality). In Central Louisiana, our highest rates for low birth weight babies, often premature and with worse outcomes are Avoyelles (11%), Catahoula (12%) and Concordia (14%). Considerable success has been achieved in Central Louisiana, which achieved infant mortality of 4.7/1,000 in 2015, well below state and national rates; it rebounded to 8.3/1,000 in 2017, a discouraging increase. Nonetheless, the three-year average in CENLA from 2014 t0 2106 still remained the lowest in the state among the nine public health regions.

The Fetal-Infant Mortality Review and Child Death Review, as well as the associated Community Action and Advisory Team, meet on successive months in each Public Health Region in the state to examine infant deaths and explore and enhance programs to reduce them. All sudden and unexpected infant death cases are reviewed, with input from medical and non-medical personnel with expertise in different fields. Over 75 Sudden Unexplained Infant Deaths (SUIDS) occur in Louisiana each year and represent around 35% of all post-neonatal deaths. Around a quarter of such cases are "Accidental Strangulation and Suffocation in Bed" (ASSB), while around two thirds are "Sudden Infant Death Syndrome" (SIDS) cases, unexplained after autopsy and review.

Co-sleeping with adults and subsequent suffocation represents a recurrent cause of preventable infant deaths. It is not the only contributing factor, however, with many more including: very young (or old) mothers, smoking, other substance abuse, inadequate pre-natal care, poor social supports and low socio-economic and educational status. Since the causes of such deaths are legion, the responses are multifactorial. As with many health outcomes, the triad of low income, low education and low socio-economic status plays a predominant role.

Louisiana has a number of programs intended to address our unacceptable numbers of infant deaths. They include the Nurse Family Partnership (which sends visiting nurses to first time high risk mothers), New Beginnings with Volunteers of America (pregnancy testing, Medicaid applications centers, pregnancy education), Partners for Healthy Babies (connecting moms and babies to resources), Caring Choices (mental health services for addiction), United Way (resource guide for CENLA), Louisiana Breast Feeding Coalition (encouraging breast feeding with Ban the Bag and Baby Friendly Hospitals), 39 Week Delivery Policies, and various prenatal care programs (encouraged through HealthyLouisiana, as well as electronic health record use with meaningful and performance improvement measures.)

In short, the efforts and resources being deployed come from both private and public initiatives, all destined to reduce the devastating toll of infant deaths, so abundantly documented by the March of Dimes, Kid's Count and America's Health Rankings. We cannot be discouraged by the severity, complexity or historical duration of the issue of infant mortality. Parents, grandparents, health care workers, social workers and even law enforcement all need to continue the fight to end preventable infant deaths.

Partners for Health Babies: www.1800251Baby.org (1-800-251-BABY (2229))

Volunteers of America (Central Louisiana): www.voanorthla.org (318-442-8026)

Nurse Family Partnership: www.nursefamilypartnership.org (318-487-5262)

Louisiana SIDS/Safe Sleep Campaign: www.giveyourbabyspace.com

United Way Resource Guide: www.guidetohumanservices.org

Louisiana Breast Feeding Coalition: www.louisianabreastfeeding coalition.org

March of Dime: www.marchofdimes.com/pnhec/pnhec.asp

Louisiana WIC Program: http://www.dhh.louisiana.gov/index.cfm/page/ 942 or call your local Health Unit

ORGAN DONATION IN THE ELDERLY: RECIPIENTS AND DONORS

With the graying of America (100 million over 50 years old and growing) and improvements in medical techniques, the issue of organ donation in the elderly has become increasingly important. Many organs can and are being transplanted, including kidneys (16,000), livers (6,000), hearts (2,000), and lungs (1,800) in 2012 alone. Other transplantable organs or tissues include pancreases, intestines, corneas, veins, bones, bone marrow, heart valves, skin and even faces and limbs. Total organ transplants in the U.S. rose from 28,000 in 2012 to 33,600 in 2016.

Since 1982, there have been over 420,000 organ transplants (notably of kidneys, hearts, livers, lungs, pancreases and intestines). With the aging population, however, the need only becomes greater. Of the 120,000 Americans on the National Organ Waiting List, there are over 53,000 seniors between 50 and 64 years of age and 23,000 over 65. Among those on this list, 87,000 of them are waiting for a kidney and only 17,000 will receive one, while 4,600 will die waiting. The demand for kidneys is particularly acute in the African-American community, which represents 37% of those on dialysis, but only 19% of kidney recipients and only 15% of the general population.

So why does this concern the elderly population in particular? First, as mentioned above, over half of those on the National Organ Waiting List are seniors (75% are 50 years old or older). Second, in 2011, 60% of all organ recipients were over 50. Third, only 32% of donors were in this same age group. Unfortunately, since only one third of donors are over 50, but two-thirds of the recipients are in this age group, and over 75% of those waiting for organs are seniors, there is an obvious discrepancy between supply and demand in this age group.

This collision between growing organ demand and fairly flat donations creates difficult medical and ethical dilemmas. While organ allocations have long been for "the sickest first" and "those longest on the waiting lists," this practice skews the recipients toward the growing elderly population whose life expectancies are shorter and whose complication rates are higher. The United Network of Organ Sharing (UNOS) develops standards for organ transplants and has been pondering changes that would, at least in part, direct younger organs to younger recipients. Although this may smack of the dreaded "R" word ("Rationing,") the fact remains that organ transplant needs vastly exceed the demand and it appears this will only get worse in the future. Giving organs to those most likely to benefit from them over a longer time period makes intellectual (if not necessarily emotional) sense.

One obvious solution to the organ crisis is to increase the number of donors, especially in those over 50 years of age, and certainly in minority populations. Even though 20% of those over 65 believe that they are "too old to donate an organ," it is not true! The oldest kidney donor was 90 years old, and age alone does not make one ineligible. The choice to accept organ donations from living (or deceased) donors varies between medical institutions and is an organ-specific and donor-specific decision. That being said, 75% of transplant centers do not accept kidney donations from living donors 70 years old and above. Underlying medical conditions, such as diabetes, heart disease, sickle cell, liver disease or even HIV, may or may not be contraindications to donation. While the survival of transplanted organs does diminish with the age of the donor, that fact should not be reason senior citizens fail to donate.

While the topic of organ donation is very complicated, signing up to be a donor is not. If you go to www.organdonor.gov, you will be directed to your respective State Organ and Tissue Registry. The "50-Plus Campaign" specifically targets potential senior donors. You can also seek information on Donate Life America. Increasing the number of organ donors, especially seniors, is critical to closing the gap between the ever increasing needs and the limited donor pool.

www.organdonor.gov
www.donatelifeamerica.com

POVERTY AND THE ELDERLY: HEALTH IMPLICATIONS

The Kaiser Family Foundation does a state-by-state analysis of poverty in the United States among seniors. There is a "Traditional Method" of determination, and a "Supplemental Poverty Measure," each of which gives a different value, the latter being significantly higher. "Supplemental Poverty Measures" adjusts expenditures by taking local housing prices into considerations as well as factoring in job-related expenses, taxes on income and out-of-pocket expenses on health care. Not surprisingly, considerably more seniors fall in the "poverty" and the low income group (less than 200% of poverty) with the "Supplemental" than with the "Traditional Method."

Based on the 2009-2011 population surveys and using the "Supplemental Poverty measure", around 48% of all seniors live beneath the 200% of poverty level (as opposed to "only" 34% with the "Traditional Method.") One in seven seniors (15%) are below poverty (with the Supplemental Method), while those with "low income" (between 100 and 200% poverty) represent 33% of seniors. Over 50% of seniors are below 200% of poverty in 10 states, including Louisiana (with 52%), Mississippi (51%), and Georgia (54%). In Louisiana, around 19% of seniors live in poverty (15% by the "Traditional Method.")

Since money reputedly buys neither health nor happiness, why is this important? It has been well demonstrated that those with low incomes spend a disproportionate amount on health care (for those less than 200% poverty, over 50% spend at least 20% of their income on health care). The same holds true with housing where around 20% of those in poverty spend up to 60% of their income for housing, a number that increases with those paying a mortgage.

When poor seniors spend 60% on housing and 20% on health care, it leaves little for other basic necessities such as utilities and food. Around 22% of low-income elderly reported food insecurity (as "low" or "very low" food security already in 2008.) When fresh fruits and vegetables are either unavailable (as occurs in low-income "food deserts") or too costly, cheap, unhealthy, processed foods become stables leading to overt obesity and undiagnosed nutritional deficiencies. This decreases immunity and increases susceptibility to infections, complicating an already difficult health situation. Two thirds of seniors have one chronic disease and see up to seven doctors. This rises to as high as 20% who have five chronic disease and see up to 14 physicians (often very expensive sub-specialists).

With 10,000 Americans a day turning 65, the increase in the elderly population, especially those in poverty or with low incomes, becomes a tidal wave of predictable needs. The National Retirement Risk Index (predicting those unlikely to have enough money to maintain their standard of living) rose from 44 to 53 percent from 2007 to 2010. This corresponds with a similar result from the Elder Economic Security Initiative (EESI). As previously mentioned, over 50% of seniors are currently "economically insecure" (below 200% poverty level).

Increasing medical needs are coupled with a leveling off of health-related expenditures, which still account for 18% of the U.S. gross domestic product, or about 3 trillion dollars a year, already an unsustainable amount. Increases in the cost of technology and pharmaceuticals add to the perfect storm that already threatens to submerge our elderly poor and soon-to-be-poor.

Although it has been said that "the poor you shall always have among you," we have both a moral and medical obligation to make sure that poverty does not translate into morbidity and that our most vulnerable citizens receive the care they need.

SOCIAL CAPITAL AND HEALTH
IN THE ELDERLY

Dr. Robert Putnam used the concept of "social capital" in his groundbreaking book, "***Bowling Alone in America***." Social capital can loosely be defined as the "glue that binds people together." More technically, it included measures of (1) "Community Organizational Life," (2) "Engagement in Public Life," (3) "Community Volunteerism," (4) "Informal Sociability" and (5) "Social Trust." These measures deal with levels of community social engagement. What exactly does this have to do with health in the elderly?

In fact, Dr. Putnam was able to demonstrate a tight correlation between the strength of a state's "Social Capital Index" and a number of other health-related indices for adults. In other words, the lower the Social Capital Index, the lower the results for a state's health outcomes, educational performance, longevity and even its tolerance for racial and gender equality. Although Dr. Putnam did not establish a direct cause and effect relationship, the correlations are astonishing.

Louisiana, as a state, ranks very low in its Social Capital Index along with its neighbors states, Mississippi and Alabama. In fact, the entire Old South ranked lower than states in the Mid-West, East or West. It also remains true that increasing social capital is associated with better health outcomes. From an individual perspective, enhancing social capital can be as easy as volunteering, voting in elections, inviting friends over to dinner and demonstrating more tolerance for those different from us. While Louisianans are very social, sociability tends to split along lines of race, income and religion, or in other words, "birds of a feather flock together." This is what Dr. Putnam calls "bonding social capital" among similar individuals. The maximum improvements in personal and community health, however, come in increasing "bridging social capital" by associating and interacting with those who do not share our color, religion or income.

The paradox is that none of Mr. Putnam's measures in the Social Capital Index have anything to do with our attitudes toward health or education, but rather reflect our relationships with those around us in the larger community. We should all seek every opportunity to engage socially and to stretch our limits beyond our comfort zones. Volunteer, vote, and serve on a committee and invite people to your home, especially those beyond your personal families, churches or country club. Doing so will improve your quality of life as well as your physical and mental health. As a bonus, it will improve community health outcomes as well.

SPRINT (SYSTOLIC BLOOD PRESSURE INTERVENTION TRIAL): IMPLICATIONS FOR SENIORS

Heart disease remains the number one killer of Americans and high blood pressure (BP), a leading contributor to cardiovascular deaths, affects over a billion people worldwide. In an effort to establish the optimal treatment levels for BP in those over 50 years, Dr. Paul Whelton from Tulane University spearheaded the Systolic Blood Pressure Intervention Trial (SPRINT). This landmark study came to an early end when results revealed important benefits of aggressive blood pressure control in senior citizens. The study design included over 9,000 subjects (at 102 clinical centers throughout the United States) over the age of 50 with systolic blood pressures between 130 and 180. Those with previous strokes, congestive heart failure, renal failure (with our without polycystic kidney disease) and diabetes were excluded from the trial.

Subjects were randomized to either a "standard treatment" or "intensive treatment," the latter having a systolic BP goal of 120 or less. End points included heart attack (MI), stroke, congestive heart failure (CHF), cardiovascular (CV) related death and all-cause mortality. The study was stopped almost two years earlier than its 5-year end point because there was already a significant reduction in heart attacks, congestive heart failure, cardiovascular and all-cause mortalities in the intensively treated group. In fact there was a 25% reduction in CV deaths and a 27% reduction in all-cause mortalities among those with "intensive" treatment.

In the aggressively treated group, there were some side effects, including an increased number of subjects with low serum sodium and potassium levels, as well as increased episodes of orthostatic hypotension (dizziness with changes of position). Nonetheless, it appears that the benefits of more aggressive treatment of systolic BPs in senior citizens still outweigh the risks.

Even though, as mentioned, diabetics (and those with kidney failure or prior stroke) were excluded from the trial, the results imply that stricter BP control in those over 50 years of age is both achievable and beneficial. This contradicts recommendations from the 8th Joint National Committee (JNC 8) that recommended higher acceptable BP values in older Americans (up to 150 systolic). The SPRINT results, however, will surely be incorporated into future discussions for the next set of BP guidelines (JNC 9). And the 130/80 thresholds may become the new gold standard. The American Heart Association has already set their goal of 130/80 for all adults, including seniors, although other national organizations have not modified their higher goals as of now.

If lower BP benefits older Americans, does this also hold true for the almost 10% of adult Americans with diabetes (many of them over 50)? That question, as well as the effects of lower systolic blood pressures on cognition and renal function, remains to be determined.

Now, with the landmark SPRINT findings available, the threshold of treatment of blood pressure in senior citizens, and perhaps all Americans, should drop much lower. Hopefully mortality statistics for older Americans will drop correspondingly and we will make another dent in the huge number of those who die from our number one killer, heart disease.

STATINS: A SECOND LOOK FROM THE U.S. PREVENTIVE SERVICES TASK FORCE

Cardiovascular disease (CVD) still remains the leading cause of death and illness in the United States today, resulting in the deaths of one third of Americans. This huge cause of morbidity and mortality has, fortunately, been steadily dropping over the last three decades (falling by around 30% from the 1980's), largely due to decreased smoking, better blood pressure control and the increased use of statins. Although the epidemic of obesity risks wiping out some of these hard-won gains, we have still made considerable progress and hope to make more in the future.

The use of statins (medications that reduce cholesterol production by inhibiting certain enzymes used in their internal production) has been very successful. There has been constant research into determining when and how much of these medications should be used. The U.S. Preventive Services Task Force (USPSTF) recently revisited the existing data to offer new recommendations. The USPSTF grades their recommendations from "A" (High certainty of substantial benefit) down to "I" (Insufficient evidence) with "B", "C" and "D" in between.

The USPSTF gives a "B" recommendation (High certainty of moderate benefit) for the use of low-to-moderate statins for the prevention of CVD in those who are (1) 40-75 years old; (2) with one or more CVD risk factors (dyslipidemia, diabetes, hypertension or smoking); and (3) with a 10% or greater 10-year risk of a cardiovascular event. The recommendation drops to a "C" (Moderate certainty of small benefit) for those with a slightly lower calculated risk (from 7.5 to 10%). Their recommendation drops to an "I" (Insufficient Evidence) for those over 76 years of age.

These recommendations require some explanation for the general public. First, the "risk factors" include "dyslipidemia" (or abnormal serum lipid levels) of an LDL-C (or "bad cholesterol") of 130 mg/dl or more, or a HDL-C (or "good cholesterol") of 40 mg/dl or less. Subjects with high "bad cholesterol" (LDL) levels (greater than 190) were excluded from the study since they are known to be at high risk and should be on statins anyway.

The risk percentage is calculated using the American College of Cardiology/American Heart Association Pooled Cohort Equations that take into consideration many factors including age, sex, race, cholesterol levels, blood pressure, anti-hypertensive treatment, diabetes and smoking status. The risk calculator tends to overestimate risk according to some critics, but is the only calculator that has been validated. Age plays a disproportionate part in the calculation, with 41% of men and 27% of women who are sixty to sixty-nine years of age having a risk of 10% or greater, regardless of other factors.

Older individual (over 75 years old) received an "I" (Insufficient Evidence) recommendation because there is so little data on primary prevention in this age group. Almost half of individual greater than 75 are already on a medication for cholesterol and most of these (80% or more) are using a statin. When individuals are over 85, the use of statins is considered of questionable value because of limited life expectancy and a lower benefit/risk ratio.

Although much of this may appear highly technical and perhaps difficult to understand, the fact remains that statin use is clearly beneficial in many individual from 40 to 75 years of age, some of whom may not be currently taking them. Underuse of statins at a low-to-moderate dose is particularly apparent in women (used by 30% of men vs. 26% of women), Blacks and Hispanics (used by 30% of Whites vs. 24% of Blacks and only 21% of Hispanics) and those without insurance (used by 48% of those with Medicare, but only 8% with no insurance.)

The choice of which statin will depend on cost, tolerance and availability, among other things. Some statins are available on $4 plans at major retail pharmacies, so cost should almost never be a limiting factor. A serious discussion with your doctor and a prescription for this miracle medication may prolong your life. Of course, smoking cession, blood pressure control and weight loss are additional critical factors in reducing cardiovascular risk.

HEALTH OUTCOMES

PARISH (COUNTY) HEALTH RANKINGS FOR CENLA & NATCHITOCHES (2017)

Every spring, the Robert Wood Johnson Foundation publishes their "County Health Rankings." This report exams every parish in Louisiana and ranks them according to their "Health Outcomes" and "Health Factors." "Health Outcomes" include measures of morbidity and mortality such as premature death, low birth weight, and days of poor physical and mental health (as reported by the person). "Health Factors" (sometimes called "Health Determinants") include a wide variety of indicators including "Health Behaviors" (such as smoking, obesity, inactivity, drinking, STDs and teen birth) and "Clinical Care" (including uninsured rates, availability of providers, preventable hospital stays and screening tests for diabetes and breast cancer). Health Factors also include "Social and Economic Factors," notably high school graduation rates, poverty, violent crime rates, injury deaths and single-parent households. Lastly, health factors include elements of the "Physical Environment," such as air pollution, drinking water violations, housing and long commutes.

As you see, the multiple factors that result in the health outcomes demonstrate a cause and effect relationship, with poorer factors (determinants) generally resulting in worse outcomes. So how do parishes in Central Louisiana stack up against others in the state? As far as outcomes are concerned, results show that there are three separate groups: those with the best outcomes (LaSalle 16/64, Vernon 17/64 and Grant 20/64), a middle group (Rapides 36/64, Natchitoches 38/64, Avoyelles 41/64 and Winn 44/64), and a lower tier (Catahoula 58/64 and Concordia 61/64). This stratification has held true for many years, with the unhealthiest

103

parishes being along the Mississippi River, a distinction they share with counties on the other side of the river.

Since health factors and health outcomes are so closely related, you would expect a similar grouping for health factors. For the most part, that does hold true, but not completely. LaSalle (17/64), Rapides (18/64), Vernon (20/64) and Grant (24/64) fall in the best category for health factors, while Natchitoches (41/64) and Winn (47/64) fall in the middle. Once again, the Mississippi River parishes of Avoyelles (53/64), Catahoula (57/64) and Concordia (59/64) have the lowest health factors, correlating with their equally poor outcomes. This being said, Avoyelles has better outcomes than would be predicted by their health factors, while Rapides has worse outcomes than would be predicted by their factors.

What is obvious from looking at these statistics is their stability over time, with only a few positive trends. Grant has improved its health factors, as have LaSalle and Vernon Parish. There have also been improvements in outcomes in Grant (probably related to increased access to care.) Otherwise, both factors and outcomes appear to be rather static, notably for Natchitoches Parish and not unlike Louisiana's national health rankings.

While there is merit in looking at individual parishes (or counties) within individual states, it is important to put these statistics in the context of Louisiana's results when compared with other states. Alas, in the latest America's Health Rankings, Louisiana ranked 49/50 overall, with 47/50 in outcomes and 49/50 in health determinants (factors). While we have a host of poor results (40/50 or worse for obesity, inactivity, smoking, chlamydia rates, occupational deaths, violent crime, lack of insurance, and preventable hospitalizations, among others), we have very good rankings for adolescent vaccinations (12/50 or better) for meningococcus and Tdap (tetanus, diphtheria and pertussis). Vaccinations have always been a Louisiana bright spot, mostly related to LINKS (Louisiana Immunization Network for Kids) and our strict "no shots, no school" policies. Such favorable statistics for one aspect of health prove that improvements can be made with the proper programs, policies and adequate investments. Louisiana is not doomed to be last in health outcomes.

Another bright spot for Central Louisiana is its very low infant mortality rates. CENLA (OPH Region VI not including Natchitoches Parish) boasted a rate of 4.7 infant deaths/1,000 live births in 2015, the lowest in Louisiana and lower than the national rate of 5.9/1,000. CENLA's rate was also far less than the Louisiana state rate of 7.7/1,000. Sadly, our infant mortality rate in CENLA rose to 8.3/1,000 live births in 2016. Despite this rise, CENLA's 2014-2016 average remained the state's lowest (6.3/1,000 live births) among the nine public health regions.

This remarkable achievement might have many explanations, but our CENLA health units have among the highest coverage of contraceptive needs among all state parishes (over 23% satisfaction of needs and higher than state goal of 20 %.) We also have the busiest health unit (Rapides Parish) in the state, thanks to our dedicated staff and consistent parish support. Our Fetal-Infant Mortality and Child Death Reviews (under the inspired leadership of Lisa Norman) bring together a great group of partners in many disciplines related to maternal and child care. Our robust Nurse Family Partnership also contributes to this success. Natchitoches Parish in OPH Region VIII (Northwest Louisiana) lagged behind in infant mortality with regional rate of 9.0/1,000 live births, higher than both national (5.9) and state (7.7) rates for 2015.

Our state and parish statistics often hide tragic disparities in outcomes between groups based on income and education (often complicated by race). Health providers, policy makers and civic leaders in all locations should target these disparities, as persistent as they have been, for elimination. Let's hope we can build on our strengths and continue to improve health factors and their resulting health outcomes. Partnerships and persistence will help us raise our regional and state rankings so Louisiana will no longer be located at the bottom of the health statistical barrel.

REFLECTIONS ON HEALTH
OUTCOMES DISPARITIES

What are health outcome disparities? A disparity exists when the difference in outcomes cannot be attributed to some inherent genetic disposition of the affected population.

An example of genetic diseases peculiar to a certain racial group is Sickle Cell disease among Blacks or the presence of several serious metabolic disorders (such as Tay-Sachs disease) among Ashkenazi Jews (those from Eastern Europe). Despite such racial differences, attributable to genetic variations, human beings are far more alike than they are different and differences in health outcomes can be attributed to social causes far more than to biological ones.

There are no biological reasons that Black men and women die on an average 4 or 5 years earlier than Whites. There are no biological differences that cause Black babies to die twice as frequently as White babies or Black mothers to die more frequently in childbirth than White mothers. There are no biological differences that mandate three quarters of HIV/AIDS cases to be in Blacks in Louisiana, where they represent only a third of the general population.

The persistence of huge disparities in health outcomes covers an astonishing range of issues: life expectancy, cancer death rates, murder rates, infant mortality, maternal mortality, STD and HIV/AIDS rates, cardiovascular death rates, obesity rates (and closely related diabetes rates) and even hospital readmission rates. Some of these negative differences are more than double in the Black community compared to Whites and none of them have a genetic or biological basis.

The stubborn persistence of such disparities, often closely linked with low educational attainment and poverty, poses a huge challenge to those in the medical field in general, and in public health in specific. Public health deals with populations, and usually not with individuals. As such, there is a medical and moral responsibility to tackle such disparities whenever they are identified. While there is much heated discussion about the origins and responsibilities of such differences, often attributed to our history of slavery and subsequent institutional racism, they remain painful markers of a failure to achieve health equity in the United States.

What can and should be done? Firstly, health care providers and policy makers must honestly recognize the existence of such grievous differences in health outcomes. Secondly, they must be willing to make their elimination a priority. While this sounds straightforward, the association of health disparities with race and underlying social determinants (i.e. education and income) makes it much more of challenge since it affects policies in many aspects of life and not just in the limited scope of medical care alone. Thirdly, having recognized the problem and having made it a priority, health care providers and policy makers much cooperate and devote adequate resources to addressing health disparities and their root social causes.

We should all remember the immortal words of Dr. Martin Luther King, Jr. "Of all the forms of inequality, injustice in health care is the most shocking and inhumane." Health disparities are a symptom of a "social disease" resulting in unequal outcomes. Disparities should be approached this way by anyone and everyone dealing not only with health care, but also with all aspects of the society that contribute to their shameful persistence. As Malcolm X stated, "You are part of the solution or you are part of the problem."

There is no easy solution, but making the elimination of health disparities a priority should be a personal and public goal, especially for public health. When Blacks and Whites have the same life expectancy, the same infant and maternal mortality, the same STD/HIV rates and the same cancer death rates as Whites, we will know we will achieved the illusive dream of an equitable society.

SENIOR HEALTH REPORT FOR LOUISIANA (2018)

In conjunction with America's Health Rankings, there is a specific annual report issued for senior health for each state. America's Health Rankings Senior Report for 2018 is the most recent one available and it usually parallels health rankings for Louisiana as a whole, with some exceptions.

Once again, Louisiana did not rank high for its Senior Health Report. In fact we had an overall ranking of 50/50 states. The ranking is divided into two sections, "Determinants" (or factors that determine health outcomes) and "Outcomes." Although we are 43/50 for outcomes compared to other states, we ranked 50/50 for our determinants. Determinants (or health factors as they are sometimes called) help to predict future outcomes. Being last in determinants does not bode well for the future.

How do our results look and what do they mean? Health determinants are divided into behaviors, community and environmental factors, policy and clinical care. Let's focus on those areas that most need improvement (ranking of 40/50 states or worse). Our worst senior behaviors are smoking (46/50), obesity (49/50), physical inactivity (44/50) and low dental visits (48/50) and high dental extractions (44/50). Negative results for community and environmental factors include poverty (48/50), low volunteerism (50/50), poor nursing home quality (50/50) and food insecurity (49/50). Low policy factors include inadequate geriatricians (46/50). Low ranks for clinical care include low number of preventive care visits (40/50), low flu shot rates (48/50) and preventable hospitalizations (47/50).

When combined, all of these low factors (or determinants) contribute to poor health outcomes. These poor outcomes include high numbers of hip fractures (42/40), frequent mental distress (48/50), high premature deaths (43/50), frequent mental distress (48/50) and few seniors reporting good health (44/50).

Are there any bright spots in this dark picture? In fact, we have a few, with lots of home health workers (9/50), infrequent falls (30/50) and low senior drinking (22/50).

Although it was not the object of the report, the close association between low incomes, low educational level and poor health continues to haunt Louisiana. Our reputation as a "happy state" belies the fact that our happiness may be rooted in a poor understanding of our numerous health shortcomings. Everyone knows senior citizens who are happy, healthy and even wealthy, but there are huge numbers that are not. Ignorance about our health outcomes should not equate with bliss.

As a society, we can work to improve the health status of our most vulnerable citizens (both the very young and very old), especially by improving their economic and educational prospects. Our investments in youth education and job training will reap dividends for our elderly both now and in the future. The best treatment is always prevention, so we need to look upstream for the causes of so many ills that beset our elderly citizens and act accordingly.

THE WELL-BEING OF YOUNG WOMEN IN THE U.S.

Policy makers and the public expect that our well-being should increase with each successive generation. The U.S. Population Reference Bureau studies these changes and recently concentrated specifically on the well-being of young women.

They compared women in four cohorts (groups): Those born from 1930-1945, the Baby Boomers born between 1946-1964, Gen Xers born between 1965-1981 and Millennials born from 1982-2002. Fourteen separate measures were explored in an effort to answer the question of whether younger generation women are doing better or worse than their predecessors.

As usual, there was good news and bad news. There were progressive improvements in reduced high school dropout rates, increased college education, reductions in the female-male wage gap, increased business ownership, decreased cigarette smoking and increased female representation in government.

Unfortunately, the bad news leaves considerable room for reflection and improvement. The Millennials have less women in high paying STEM occupations, while the percent of Millennial women living in poverty has increased to 16.9%. Unemployment increased from Gen-Xers to Millennials as has maternal mortality. Other sad indicators of decreased well-being have been increases in suicide and incarceration rates among Millennials. Within these negative criteria are persistent racial disparities with worse outcomes among Blacks, Hispanics and Native Americans compared to Whites.

Policy makers and healthcare providers alike should be gladdened by the improvements, but also disturbed by the stalled or worsening trends. While suicides increased from a low of 4.4/100,000 to 6.3/100,000, overdose rates skyrocketed from 2.9 to 12.5/100,000 over the same time period, a fourfold increase. Equally disturbing are the incarceration rates among young women, which rose ten times since the 1970's even though crime rates plateaued or even decreased.

Millennials act a bit like canaries in the coal mine. Their outcomes should serve as a warning and a wake-up call to the public and policy makers. We must also continue to focus on persistent, corrosive disparities between Black and Hispanic women and White women in our quest to achieve a healthier, more equitable society. Our young women (and men) deserve no less. Increased well-being from generation to generation should be the norm and not the exception.

HEALTHCARE POLICY

REFLECTIONS ON THE FINANCIAL STABILITY OF THE LOUISIANA OFFICE OF PUBLIC HEALTH

Reduction in health disparities is a constant theme across public health departments throughout the United States. There is a general understanding among those involved with public health that "there is no health equity without social equity." The federal government has many initiatives, which may or may not be mirrored at the state and local level. Universal health insurance, by whatever mechanism, has been a long-standing goal of the public health community (variably appreciated by local or state entities.) It has also been a goal of all other developed countries, which have achieved it through national programs of one form or another. The United States alone distinguishes itself by pouring massive amounts of money into healthcare (18% of the GDP or over $3 trillion dollars annually) with a persistent elevated percentage of uninsured (around 9%, down from 14% pre-Obamacare) and many more underinsured, with corresponding mediocre health outcomes. Our current national (and state debate) reflects continued controversies, long resolved elsewhere in the developed world.

The current role of public health in Louisiana centers on those "traditional" services (i.e. vaccinations, reproductive health, disease surveillance with sexually transmitted diseases and tuberculosis, children's special health services, WIC, disaster preparedness, etc.). It should also include those broader public health goals of education, alignment of citizens with services, advocacy for health issues, creating partnerships, etc. For better or worse, "public health is, by its very nature, political." There are almost unavoidable tensions between short-term political cycles and long-term public health outcomes.

Numerous initiatives exist, both public and private, to examine data and use it to achieve better health outcomes. The Kaiser Foundation, Robert Wood Johnson Foundation, March of Dimes and their affiliated products (America's Health Rankings, County Health Rankings, Kids Count and others) all have programs designed to mobilize local communities and state organizations to focus on strategic issues. We do not have to re-invent the wheel, but rather we need to seek out existing opportunities to align ourselves with larger initiatives. Attempts to do so must be encouraged and recognized to insure innovation. They also require a maximization of stakeholder participation, including clients, and process transparency in order to produce successful outcomes.

Why is achieving better health outcomes so difficult, especially in the Southern states? Health is really a by-product of other factors. It is a dependent variable and not an independent variable. Improved health comes from improvements in education, income and social status, three sides of a triangle, with health as its delineated area. Thus, when any of these three elements improve, health outcomes improve accordingly. When the elements increase together, the area in the triangle (health) improves at a maximal rate (the area of an isosceles triangle is greatest.) It helps to improve any of the sides of the triangle (i.e. income, education and socio-economic status) independently, but the biggest bang for your buck is when all three increase simultaneously. Louisiana's problem is that there are many "small triangles" and not enough "large triangles." Also, improving education, income and social status seem to fall outside of the normal focus of public health (with the exception of education.)

So what is to be done? The situation of healthcare providers varies wildly from region to region. It seems unlikely that a one-size-fits-all approach for public health will be successful or even practical. Regions should be given the ability to find local solutions, working with existing partners and personnel. Solutions may take different forms in different areas and that diversity should be accepted and encouraged. If the state is determined to get out of the direct care delivery business, then that should be the clearly stated goal. Accordingly, every opportunity to encourage local alternative providers, where they exist, should be sought out and implemented. Because of the complexity of the issues and the diversity within the state, all projects must be timed appropriately and, as mentioned earlier, maximize participation of stakeholder groups while making the process (necessarily messy) as transparent as possible. What you do "with people" has a much better chance of long-term success than what you do "to people."

Financial stability depends on two factors: state funded support and internally generated revenues. Because of the nature of our services and the population served (largely Medicaid), public health cannot be financially independent. Public health will never pay for itself. There will always be some level of public funding required, whether it is state or federal. Despite that fact, there are still enormous opportunities for increasing revenue. Within the state agencies, there was a long-standing pernicious attitude that revenue "did not matter." Of course money matters, especially when public funding has been so drastically reduced. The absence of electronic health records delayed improvements. Billing has also been terrifically complicated by the HealthyLouisiana (formerly BayouHealth) Medicaid managed care initiative, which multiplied the number of denials. That being said, OPH must devote adequate resources to maximizing billing and handling the huge volume of denials. FQHC's have recognized this problem and put specialized individuals in each FQHC to handle these complications, with successful results. The other barrier to stability is the uncertainty surrounding long-term funding from the public sector. Commitment to public health should be clearly and credibly stated to alleviate the constant anxiety in the field. It remains difficult to motivate OPH employees who doubt the long-term stability of their positions. This is especially true with performance improvement initiatives that are neither linked to increased income nor job security. Participation of local governments has also been subject to unpredictable changes and competing priorities, often at the expense of pubic health funding.

Current initiatives to increase reimbursement rates have taken place at a state and regional level. In Region VI (Central Louisiana), we have consistently reinforced the importance of seeing clients, not canceling clinics, billing all appropriate clients, and collecting money through the new electronic health system. The results have been apparent from a collection standpoint. The move toward electronic health records should be continued at an accelerated rate with the best possible system available for a reasonable price.

In Central Louisiana, we have also remained flexible and the former Regional Nursing Supervisor (an APRN) and the Regional Administrator/ Medical Director have actively participated in Reproductive Health Clinics for cross-coverage purposes. We worked to increase the number of Reproductive Health clinics and both the Regional Nursing Supervisor and the Regional Medical Director perform regular clinic duties in collaboration with parish nursing personnel. This enhances Reproductive Health services in Region VI (already the highest in the state despite one of the lowest population bases) and the highest number of services per capita of any OPH Region. Increased services translate into enhanced OPH revenues even though OPH can never hope to be self-supporting.

In order to enhance productivity, more resources must be devoted to the question of handling billing denials. There needs to be an alignment of incentives between the Electronic Health Record system and OPH. A Regional Administrative Manager (RAM) should be present in all OPH Regions given the critical nature of that position. The RAM is the best person to handle billing, implementation of electronic health records, denials and other large-scale projects of critical importance in close collaboration with Central Office. Recovery of denials should pay for their positions or that of similar individuals at the state level.

Many public health departments nationwide are struggling with decreased funding, shifting mandates, negative public perceptions, hostile legislatures and all sorts of other issues. Since the reality varies from state to state, responses to these challenges are as varied as health departments. To confound the issue, Louisiana has a state-driven system that is regionalized, a situation that is rare. Most health departments have county health commissions that are funded by local taxes. Louisiana, with its Local Governing Entities (i.e. Human Service Districts) is pushing in that direction. Shifting the responsibilities to the locals is certainly understandable, but only if the funding is also guaranteed. Much as with poor vs. rich counties (or parishes), when the responsibilities are dispersed, the income may not be, so the rich get richer while the poor go bankrupt. Retaining a state structure does allow some "sharing of the wealth" (a phrase made so famous by Huey P. Long) as well as promoting a certain standardization and oversight. Each OPH region, as mentioned, will be different, so creativity and innovation should be recognized and celebrated whenever they occur. The health problems in Louisiana, so tied to income, education and social status, and complicated by horrific racial disparities, should never be accepted as inevitable. We are up to the challenge, but accountability in the field and administrative support and leadership from Baton Rouge must be forthcoming. Leadership in the field is also critical. Personnel will work for leaders they believe in with far more enthusiasm than for abstract notions of "the public good" or "quality improvement."

OPH will be working together in periodic meetings, some of them in conjunction with future public health accreditation, to develop goals, objectives and strategies to address each issue. Planning at the state level needs to be coordinated with other work being done throughout OPH. Thus, it is very important that leaders throughout OPH give their input on the responses to the issues reviewed above, particularly those in relation to strategic planning at the highest level of our centralized OPH structure. Constant communication between the OPH Regions and the central office, notably the OPH programs, remains critical to future success.

The day may come when the Louisiana OPH gets out of the direct care business and concentrates on preventive care and surveillance functions, but that day is not yet here. Considering the dearth of alternative providers and the heavy reliance by the population on OPH for safety net services, notably for reproductive health and WIC, that transition may still be far off in the future. Until that time, we can only hope to provide the best, most comprehensive and patient-oriented services possible.

MACRA, MIPPS AND APMS: COMING TO A DOCTOR NEAR YOU

Although the ACA (aka "Obamacare") may be headed for major modifications, MACRA is still coming to a doctor near you. MACRA stands for the Medicare Access and CHIP Reauthorization Act. (The acronym within an acronym is CHIP, which stands for the Children's Health Insurance Program.) MARCA is not part of the ACA and was passed by a solid bipartisan majority to improve health care outcomes and stabilize or reduce medical costs.

MACRA affects those providers who receive significant (over $30,000/year) reimbursements from CMS (Centers for Medicare and Medicaid Services), which means almost all doctors who see elderly or pediatric patients. What is MACRA and what is it supposed to do for you? First, it repeals the SGR or Sustainable Growth Rate that fixed physician reimbursement and became an annual nightmare for Congress. Second, MACRA, which will be implemented over a several year process, hopes to establish quality-based reimbursement. MACRA has two major components, MIPS (Merit-Based Incentive Payment System) and APM (Alternative Payment Models).

The former, MIPS will apply to most doctors (between 80 to 90%). It entails four performance categories: (1) Quality, (2) Resource Use (or Cost), (3) Clinical Practice Improvement Activities and (4) Advancing Care Information (formerly "Meaningful Use.") For the layperson, this complex set of criteria (which are not given equal weight) covers six quality measures (out of 300 possible), tracks medical cost per clinician, encourages quality improvement in care coordination and patient engagement, and promotes the effective use of electronic health records. The changes in relative weight in the criteria will occur over time. For example, "Quality" will be worth 60% in 2019 and drop to only 30% in 2021, while "Cost," which is not included at all in 2019, rises to 30% by 2021.

MACRA appears to be an additional complicated burden on the physician, so why would doctors be interested in participating? The motivation, besides improved patient care, comes back to money. The whole project must be "budget neutral," so over the years there will be a steady increase in payments to those doctors who successfully participate and a gradual decline (up to 9% by 2022) for those who do not. Under certain circumstances, over-achievers can increase reimbursement by anywhere from 9 to 27% with special bonuses. The intent is to drive quality up while driving cost down by rewarding the best and most efficient providers. Again, MACRA had broad bipartisan support with huge majorities in both the Senate and House when it was passed and is surely not going away.

The other payment system is Advanced Alternative Payment Models (APMs) and refers only to specific groups as determined by the Centers for Medicare and Medicaid Services (CMS). Such participants include Next Generation ACOs (or Accountable Care Organizations), Patient Centered Medical Homes, various Bundled Payment Models (Oncology Care Model and End Stage Renal Disease Care Model, for example) some Medicare Shared Savings Programs and some commercial contracts with shared risks. All these complex models include receiving financial incentives to increase quality while assuming increased financial risk.

As a patient, you will probably not see too many changes, at least not initially. But the end result should be an increase in quality, deceasing cost, and enhanced patient-physician communication through electronic means. All of this complexity is geared toward reducing the staggering $3 trillion spent annually on healthcare to achieve often-mediocre results by international standards.

Again, all of these provider-directed changes do not remove the individual responsibility to eat a healthy diet, maintain a healthy weight, exercise and refrain from self-destructive activities. You and your doctor should always be the ones to decide your course of action in a sincere dialogue, but payers can and do influence that conversation. That is, indeed, what MARCA intends to accomplish.

INCARCERATION: LOUISIANA OVERKILL?

Louisiana tops a number of lists, some good and others not so good. We boast several of the happiest U.S. cities and have the highest percentage of native-born residents of any state. We also have world-class cuisine and popular culture, notably musical. We do, however top several "bad" lists, including the nation's highest murder rate, the highest STD/HIV rates and the highest incarceration rates per capita (over 1,400/100,000, double the U.S. average of 700 and 14 times higher than European rates of 100/100,000.)

This disturbing incarceration statistic masks another sinister statistic, that 75% of the inmates are African American despite the fact that they represent only 30% of the general Louisiana population. How did it happen that we lock up more people than any other state and that most of them are Black?

The growth of the prison complex has occurred incrementally, yet represents a constant in Louisiana. Since our incarceration rate is 1,400/100,000, it means that we have around 63,000 incarcerated adults, a huge number that is equivalent to the entire population of Alexandria and half of Rapides Parish. You might say that the prison industry is flourishing. That would be true since a vast army of guards, administrators and ancillary staff find employment there. Yet this industry also comes at a huge cost, both financially and in human terms.

Mandatory sentencing laws, often dating back to the Clinton administration's "War on Drugs," as well as those relating to minors, have filled Louisiana prisons with non-violent offenders. Besides not being able to vote while in prison, a felony conviction carries with it a lifelong stigma, as well as an inability to benefit from public housing, supplemental food programs, and other government programs after release. Worse yet, most employment applications contain the check box for "Have you ever been convicted of a felony." Since this can be anything from drug possession to murder, most employers consider a prior felony to be an exclusion criterion for employment. The result becomes unemployment and recidivism among prior convicted felons leading to a high rate of re-incarceration, thus perpetuating the prison cycle.

Incarceration also creates high financial and psychological burdens for the families of prisoners. Social stigma, loss of income, impact on children and spouses, disintegration of social networks and supports, all affect the larger community, mostly in very adverse ways. Since incarceration limits income potential and possibilities of traditional education, lowering of those two critical social determinants (income and educational level) also negatively affects health.

Incarceration and its consequences can reduce life expectancy, whether directly or indirectly. In fact, Black males in the general population already live around 5 years less than White males and over 7 years less than White females. A huge contributing fact to reduced life expectancy is death among Black adolescents where homicides (rather than motor vehicle accidents as among Whites) represent the biggest cause of death.

Homicides not only reduce life expectancy through immediate deaths, but those who are incarcerated are also doomed to live shorter lives, either through execution (a small number) or because of reduced social determinants of wealth, education or social status and the resulting poorer health outcomes.

Some initiatives should be attempted to reduce incarceration rates and their social costs: (1) Mandatory sentencing should come under scrutiny, especially for non-violent crimes. (2) The age of prosecution as adults needs to been raised (and has been recently), keeping younger non-violent offenders from getting into the revolving door of prison. (3) Banning "the box" (eliminating the check box for felony convictions, at least on initial job applications) should be implemented. (4) "Rocket dockets," or expedited judicial proceedings, should be used to divert non-violent offenders from the prison system. These and other changes are being implemented in justice reforms promoted and pursued by Governor Edwards, the results of which are just now being felt in Louisiana.

Keeping young people, especially African-Americans out of prison and out of the morgue and should be a priority. Louisiana needs growth industries besides prisons. We must get out of the top of many of the bad lists; specifically incarceration rates, but also murder, infant mortality, percent of children in poverty and obesity rates as well.

For a state blessed with abundant natural resources, we must not squander our human resources by throwing them into prison. A healthy society is a well-educated and prosperous one. We cannot incarcerate ourselves to prosperity, or even to public safety. Let's find solutions to enhance the lives of all our citizens by giving them opportunities besides crime and punishment.

Addendum: Justice reform initiated by the administration of Governor John Bel Edwards has already begun to bear fruit. It appears that Louisiana's incarceration rate has dropped considerably and that we are no longer in the top position of U.S. states. This does not appear to be associated with any increase in criminality, reinforcing the notion that incarceration alone is not a deterrent to crime, nor a long-term solution to issues of criminality in general.

MEDICARE PAYMENTS TO PHYSICIANS: TOO MUCH INFORMATION OR JUST WHAT THE DOCTOR ORDERED?

U.S. expenditures on healthcare top three trillion dollars a year, or around $9,000 dollars per person per year. The Center for Medicare and Medicaid Services (CMS) pays around $77 billion to 80,000 health care providers under the Medicare Part B Fee-for-Service program.

All aspects of healthcare have increased in cost, but procedures, imaging and lab tests have increased disproportionally. In addition, there has been a massive increase in the cost of medications, notably for the "immuno-biologicals," used in oncology (cancer), ophthalmology, rheumatology, neurology and other specialties.

Costs are rarely discussed with patients, although the American College of Physicians (ACP) has encouraged physicians to discuss cost as one of many factors in considering treatments. Unfortunately, neither patients nor physicians have a clear understanding of the cost of treatments, especially given the complexity of the billing process and the discrepancies between what is billed and what is eventually received by the provider. In order to shed some light, the Centers for Medicare & Medicaid Services (CMS) chose the bold measure of publishing the data dealing with provider reimbursements. CMS also sought to "identify spending that doesn't make sense or appears wasteful or fraudulent."

Making such information public has been opposed by the American Medical Association, ostensibly because the results might be difficult to understand or misleading. The results were, nonetheless, published and are accessible to anyone interested in looking.

Around 4,000 physicians received $1 million each while 344 received $3 million or more each. In that latter group, 150 ophthalmologists received $658 million, while one ophthalmologist in Florida raked in $20 million. Florida, with its high population of retirees, dominated the states for the top paid physicians, followed by California, New Jersey, Texas and New York.

Jonathan Blum, CMS Principle Deputy Administrator warned against "jumping to conclusions," an opinion shared by the AMA. Examination of the data can, however, lead to a more rational allocation of resources. Primary care physicians, although they represent the bulk of providers and are the cornerstone of care, received only 20% of Medicare's total physician reimbursements. The average internist received $95,466, while the average cardiologist received $223,248.

While the data are subject to misinterpretation and may represent a challenge to physician for privacy concerns, as Gail Wilensky, former Medicaid Director under President G.W. Bush pointed out, "Transparency outweighs potential damage …and there should be a fast way for providers to correct errors."

CMS Data on individual providers can now be researched and include the amount they are paid, the number of Medicare beneficiaries treated and the number of services rendered. From a Medicare prospective, the priority remains "Detecting improper payments …in order to protect beneficiaries and taxpayers." It also encourages the public to become involved in the billing process rather than remaining passive observers.

Debra Ness, President of the National Partnership for Women and Families said, "I think shining the light of transparency helps everyone become more accountable and more conscious of what they are doing." So, let there be light and the truth shall set us free!

PUBLIC HEALTH AND PUBLIC RESPONSIBILITY

Public Health has a long and distinguished history with many accomplishments. As a "public function," it often benefits from a combination of federal, state and local funding. Unlike most states, Louisiana has a regionalized system with nine public health regions, each containing a variable number of parishes, but each overseen by a single Regional Administrator/Medical Director. Most state health departments are fairly limited in scope and each county has its own health department, overseen by a Board of Health (or County Health Commission) made up of local representatives.

The parish contribution to public health in Louisiana includes (but is not limited to) providing and maintaining a "health unit" (at least as far as the building itself is concerned). To this end, each parish establishes a millage (property tax) determined and approved by the citizens of that parish. There is a minimal millage requirement, but not a maximum one, and these millages vary dramatically in the amount of funds generated depending on the millage rate, the population, and the prosperity of the parish. Some parishes are much poorer and less populated than others and generate very modest revenues, while others are flush with cash.

Wording of the parish millages is very important and also varies drastically from parish to parish. Some millage wording limits expenditures to maintenance and operation of a health unit. Other millage wording allows for much more latitude and includes other "health-related activities," which might include anything from running an animal shelter, to mosquito abatement, to providing funds for parish prisoner health care.

While most employees at health units are state employees, much of the funding for their salaries comes through federal entitlement programs such as Title X (Family Planning and Reproductive Health), Title V (Maternal and Child Health Services) and the Children's Nutritional Act (Women, Infant and Children supplemental food programs.) Other federal funding, mostly from preventive block grants, covers all or part of programs and personnel dealing with sexually transmitted disease monitoring (including HIV), tuberculosis, other disease surveillance, immunizations and even disaster preparedness activities.

In Louisiana, there still remains a substantial direct health care role which may have been all or partially assumed by private providers elsewhere in the state or nation, a trend which has accelerated within the last decade. Some of those activities formerly performed by public health in Louisiana, are now mostly offered by private entities (notably federally qualified health centers) and include well child visits (Kid-Med), prenatal care, immunizations, STD treatment, WIC and contraceptive services. How many of these services are still offered by local health units varies dramatically from parish to parish. The regional Offices of Public Health still oversees disease surveillance functions for TB, STD case management, immunizations, WIC, disaster preparedness and environmental health (sanitarian and engineering activities).

In most other states, as mentioned, public health units and public health services are run and financed through county boards of health (or commissions), with little or no state funding or presence. While functional, this county-by-county approach can make services very unequal between rich and poor counties, something the Louisiana regional and centralized approach tends to mitigate.

Parishes throughout Central Louisiana have proven consistent and generous in their support of public health. Many parishes employ clerical and clinical staff in health units, not to mention janitorial staff and maintenance workers. Yet Central Louisiana also remains a region where the contribution of public health to direct patient care remains among the highest in the state. In fact, OPH Region VI (CENLA) sees more reproductive health patients per capita than another OPH Region. In addition, we are the only WIC provider in our parishes.

Of course, all health-related decisions must contain a significant component of individual responsibility. People make personal decisions about what they eat, if they smoke or not, if they have safe or unsafe sex, or whether they consume drugs and alcohol inordinately. But public policy, taxes, zoning, educational programs and funding, notably of health units, all significantly affect health outcomes as well.

When voting citizens must make the painful choice about voting for millages (taxes), remember that sometimes you really do get what you pay for. Also, remember to scrutinize health unit millage budgets, always under the supervision of elected police jury representatives, and carefully read the language of any proposed millage. This is necessary if you truly want public health services and not the diversion of funds to unrelated, non-public health activities. Public oversight and transparency are the cornerstones of good government and language really does matter both in both personal life and public health.

SARPS AND SANES: NEW HOPE FOR VICTIMS OF SEXUAL ASSAULT

Public revelations about victims of sexual assault being billed by hospitals for their forensic medical examinations resulted in indignation and the subsequent passage of Louisiana Act 229. While not perfect, the Act addressed these billing practices, as well as other inconsistencies in the current process in some areas of the state.

Act 229 clearly establishes the need for a SARP (Sexual Assault Response Plan) in each of the 9 public health regions of the state. The Act also declares that the parish coroners (or their approved delegate) are responsible for performing the forensic medical exam. These delegated providers may include emergency room doctors or what is known as SANEs (Sexual Assault Nurse Examiners.) These latter are nurses who undergo a vigorous training for such exams and are fully capable of completing the complex process of gathering information, performing the exam and collecting specimens from the victims. They also remain qualified to present the evidence in court where some cases of sexual assault inevitably end.

Parish coroners also designate the facility where the forensic exams take place. Some coroners, who are not physicians, transfer victims to more appropriate facilities, even in another parish. That being said, all ERs must perform an initial screening medical assessment to ensure that victims do not have other injuries that must be treated and stabilized prior to transfer.

Wherever the victim ends up, there should be a victim advocate available as well as a representative of law enforcement when the victim chooses to report the assault. While many victims have the right to choose whether to report or not, minors, victims of sex trafficking and those unable to give consent must have their cases reported.

Hospitals must have policies and plans to treat victims of sexual assault who cannot be billed for any services related to the forensic medical exam. This non-billing policy must be posted in the emergency room and be made available in pamphlet form to any victim.

Sexual assault kits should be standardized and most of the time will be brought to the healthcare facility by law enforcement. Some facilities keep a limited stock of kits for those victims who choose not to report at the time of the incident. The completed kits are given to law enforcement that transports them to an appropriate crime lab for analysis, after which completed kits are stored back with law enforcement. The hospitals store kits for non-reporting victims in a designated location and with a well-defined system of labeling. The hospitals and other providers, including the victim, may apply for reimbursement from the Crime Victim Compensation Fund for up to $1,000/case (a very modest sum considering the personnel costs alone.)

Regional Office of Public Health Medical Directors were mandated to coordinate the development of a regional Sexual Assault Response Plan (SARP), which includes, at very least, a list of resources for victims and current policies and practices in the parishes, including how and where assault kits are stored and transported. This plan, created with stakeholder input, will become effective on February 1 of each year and be reviewed annually.

The patchwork of policies and practices that characterized the current situation in many parts of the state should gradually give way to a far more systematic approach to sexual assault victims, who should never be penalized (or billed) in the process. For that, Act 229 comes as a welcome incentive, especially to those parishes and regions that have not had comprehensive policies and procedures. The problem of sexual assault (and domestic violence in general) remains a significant one in Louisiana and the United States. Act 229, while amenable to improvement, should provide motivation to move in the right direction for optimal treatment of sexual assault victims.

IN AND OUT OF THE HOSPITAL: AN EXPENSIVE, VEXING PROBLEM

Being admitted to the hospital can be a dramatic experience for everyone. It disproportionately involves older Americans since they are the ones most likely to be hospitalized. In order to be admitted (as opposed to being treated in the emergency room and discharged), the patient, old or young, must satisfy criteria of "intensity of service" and "severity of illness." In other words, you must be very sick and your treatment must require resources and techniques only available to inpatients.

For a decade or more, hospitals have been reimbursed for admissions based on a system of Diagnostic Related Groups (DRGs). That means that the payer (in this case CMS, the Centers for Medicare and Medicaid Services) pays only a fixed sum for a specific diagnosis, regardless of how long the hospital keeps the patient. This provides a huge monetary incentive to keep hospitalizations down to the strict minimum number of days.

There has been a proliferation of case managers working both in the emergency room and in the hospital to insure that only appropriate patients are admitted and, once admitted, that they stay the minimum time necessary.

Since short stays run the risk of not adequately treating the patient's conditions, there is also a payment disincentive (i.e. penalties) for frequent readmissions. This discourages recurrent hospitalizations that might compensate for short stays and smaller payments. These punitive measures to reduce re-hospitalizations have placed an additional burden on hospitals and hospital systems to coordinate post-hospital care and reduce re-admissions as much as possible.

As with most programs, there is always the law of unintended consequences. Since one out of five Medicare patients are re-admitted within 30 days of discharge, the total financial penalties for "avoidable" re-admissions amounted to $17 billion dollars in 2010 for three major diagnoses: congestive heart failure (CHF), pneumonia and acute myocardial infarctions (MIs). Since many hospitals, especially those in more economically challenged areas, often operate on razor-thin profit margins, this has become an object of intense anxiety and scrutiny.

G.K. Singh developed an "Area Deprivation Index" or ADI in 2003 that included 17 factors (i.e. income, education, housing, and employment), not unlike similar indices used in other countries. The ADI was used by MJH Kind et al. to establish a correlation between the ADI and re-hospitalizations (Ann Inter Med. 2014;162:756-774). They found that residence in the 15% most disadvantaged neighborhoods was a strong predictor of re-hospitalization, similar to that related to chronic pulmonary disease. The residents of the 15% most disadvantaged neighborhoods (nationally) were more likely to be black, on Medicaid and suffer from more CHF, COPD and hypertension.

In addition, the hospitals located in or near these disadvantaged neighborhoods were more likely to be "safety net hospitals," those serving mostly low-income residents, often underinsured or uninsured, and many of them elderly Medicare patients. These same hospitals shoulder the burden of higher re-hospitalization rates and the possibilities of higher CMS penalties, a double whammy.

All hospitals confront re-admissions with a variety of case management and post-hospitalization initiatives, which include assuring rapid medical follow-ups, use of home health and community health workers, and other "transitional care services." Because the socio-economic determinants underlying the disadvantage are so pervasive and multifactorial, hospitals find themselves confronted with issues of global community assessments, far outside of their usual scope of their practice (or comfort zones). Such assessments are mandated for all not-for-profit hospitals, many of which operate in low-income areas. Major hospital systems find themselves obligated to link with other community practices and providers, as well as public health departments, to offer a more holistic approach to patient care. This shift from an individual patient to a community perspective has posed huge conceptual and logistic challenges to many hospital systems.

The fact remains that where you live, at least when you live in an area of profound disadvantage, is more likely to predict your chances for re-hospitalization than the diseases from which you suffer. It requires meaningful partnerships among health providers, educators, business leaders, public health and community members to eliminate areas of "concentrated disadvantage" and consequently improve health and reduce re-hospitalizations.

STATISTICS, RATINGS AND
HALF-TRUTHS: APPLES AND ORANGES

The public often relies on various ratings from official or unofficial sources to make their choices about health care facilities and providers. Periodically, hospital ratings appear that are touted to the general public to extol the virtues of one institution or another. Determining whether these are more or less popularity contests or rigorous objective evaluations requires consumer scrutiny to determine. As the ancient Latin statement goes "*Caveat Emptor*" (Buyer Beware).

Some surveys, such as patient satisfaction surveys, may be administered to only a small sampling of individuals. Other surveys rely on self-reporting by consumers, thus making any serious conclusions almost impossible. The alert consumer is usually skeptical of such results, and with reason. The worst evaluations from a consumer perspective, however, are those that appear to be scientific and objective, yet compare apples and oranges, thus distorting the significance and meaning of the results.

A case in point might be a Five Star rating for a hospital. Although such an institution may have definite merit, a closer look causes one to ponder the significance. Hospitals, whether they are for-profit or not-for-profit, must serve the communities in which they are located. Part of that service includes a functional emergency room that, by law, cannot turn away any patients if they have a true emergency. (These are EMTALA laws that prevent hospitals from steering away non-paying patients to other institutions.) This invariably means that full-service hospitals will be treating a certain percentage of indigent and uninsured patients depending on their geographical location.

This group of uninsured or underinsured patients includes many with multiple medical problems, often long ignored and exacerbated by non-compliance. These individuals come disproportionately from low-income, low-educational level populations. This same demographic supplies a disproportionate number of people who are also re-admitted to the hospital within 30 days of discharge. Many of these people live in specific census tracts, characterized by "concentrated disadvantage," and fraught with problems associated with unfavorable social determinants (i.e. poverty, low academic achievement and low social status.)

Medical outcomes, of course, correlate directly with the type of population that is served. When a facility does not have an emergency room and most affiliated physicians do not accept uninsured or Medicaid patients, the "sampling error" for statistical significance becomes overwhelming. Non-representative sampling gives uninterruptable or grossly misleading results.

If, as an institution, you only care for those without the litany of social issues, then your results are more likely to be favorable. The non-medical term for treating only insured patients is "cherry picking." Some institutions can engage in this activity by being situated in high-income areas with few uninsured patients ("concentrated advantage"), definitely not the case in Central Louisiana. Other institutions restrict their activities by not accepted cases with the litany of social issues (uninsured and Medicaid), often the most challenging from a medical, societal and financial perspective. Either way, the institutions game the system to their advantage.

Is such patient selection illegal? No, as long the institution is fully licensed by the federal government from which it derives at least some of its income, notably through CMS (Center for Medicare and Medicaid Services). But licensure of facilities unable or unwilling to operate a full-service emergency room has become increasingly difficult and came to a screeching halt some years ago.

Licensing agencies recognized the deleterious effect of "cherry picking" on competing full-service hospitals, especially those located in low-income areas. Institutions that achieve unusually high quality ratings should be congratulated, of course. It takes careful management and planning to satisfy the criteria of rating agencies. But high rankings alone should not obscure the fact that any rating, to be meaningful, must compare apples to apples, and not apples to oranges.

While the gullible will be impressed by any positive results, astute observers should look beyond the smoke and mirrors to see how results were obtained and what population is being served with which specific services.

WHEN IS A DOCTOR TOO
OLD TO PRACTICE?

Central Louisiana, like everywhere in the United States, has a significant number of practicing physicians over 65. In the U.S., there are well over 64,000 physicians over 70 still working. Baby boomer physicians have increased from 9.4% of practicing physicians in 1985 to 15.1% in 2011, and there has been a four-fold increase since 1975.

Many American workers are aging and in some highly skilled and responsible professions, such as with airline pilots, mandatory retirement occurs at 65. In Belgium, professors, including those at the medical school, must retire at 70. Does this mean that all doctors must hang up their stethoscopes or scalpels at 70 because of inevitable loss of mental and physical prowess? Certainly not! But the question still remains, how long should a doctor practice?

Considering this a patient-safety issue, some hospitals have quietly begun to institute competency testing in one form or another when doctors reach 70. This usually includes some mental and physical screening tests, followed by more comprehensive testing if any abnormalities are identified. Preliminary testing, which can cost from $300 to $500 per physician and is paid for by the hospital, can be mandated or suggested by a peer review process. Some physicians, confronted with the prospect of "failing the test," may choose to resign, while others may have to undergo remedial training, restriction of privileges, limitation of night call, or peer review of documentation.

Such testing measures remain far from generalized and specialty medical groups have not endorsed such testing, despite exploratory discussions by the AMA. Some older physicians vehemently oppose any age-related testing. They insist, in fact, that most problem physicians are in their forties and fifties and that their issues often revolve around substance abuse and behavioral problems unrelated to age. In addition, eliminating older, highly experienced physicians from the community only aggravates national shortages of doctors, especially those doing primary care.

Many worry that across the board age-related testing might result in accusations of age discrimination and the litigation that might follow (although such lawsuits have proven uncommon). So how does a hospital balance patient-safety issues against the rights of their older physicians, many of whom are unable or unwilling to recognize their own limitations? The answer is not easily at all!

Contentious battles have broken out in various hospitals, notably Stanford Medical Center, over this very issue. Champion older physicians have refused to participate in testing and the administration capitulated rather than fire a whole group of distinguished and functional older doctors. While self-limitations sometimes work, peer evaluations on a case-by-case basis appear to be the most promising practice. Even that has its pitfalls, however, when personal vendettas and private agendas might cloud objective observations.

If your doctor is over 65, 70 or even 80, you can certainly vote with your feet if you feel they have become forgetful, irascible, unpredictable or unreliable. Remember, however, that older physicians have a wealth of experience and are less likely than their younger colleagues to be sleep-deprived, over-burdened, or consumed with ambition. They are also more likely to know the patient's history and spend more time in clinic with them, regardless of the demands of electronic health records. For the hospitals, the issue remains a burning one and will likely undergo significant developments in the not-too-distant future. Now, for patients as well as institutions, it is best to proceed with prudence on a case-by-case basis.

Page, Leigh. "Should Doctors Be Tested For Competence at Age 65?" Medscape. Http://www.medscape.com/view article/848937

HEALTH EQUITY IN LOUISIANA: THE BURDEN OF SOUTHERN HISTORY

Once again, Louisiana ranked near the bottom in the state health rankings (49/50). This dismal rank has remained virtually unchanged since 1990 when the Robert Wood Johnson Foundation began publishing America's Health Rankings.

County (or Parish) health rankings are often a more nuanced look, with parishes within Louisiana ranked from one to 64 based on health outcomes (and health factors). Some parishes do much better than others. St. Tammany Parish ranks consistently near the top while East Carroll (and other adjacent river parishes) trail far behind.

If all U.S. counties are ranked, our best (St. Tammany) falls around 600 out of 3,155 counties, while East Carroll ranks 3,150 (fifth from the bottom). So when you are the best in Louisiana, you still only make it to the top third of U.S. counties, while East Carroll scraps the bottom of the barrel.

On the one hand, there are, of course, very healthy, health-conscious individuals throughout our state. On the other hand, there is a majority who remain unhealthy and often unconcerned. Sadly, the worst outcomes in any criteria, whether it is life expectancy, infant mortality, maternal mortality, cancer deaths, diabetes, obesity, cardiovascular disease or strokes, the African-American community suffers the worst outcomes.

Such dismal statistics have little to do with genetics, but have everything to do with poverty and low educational levels, both social determinants of health. Your zip code, or where you live and under what circumstances have more impact on health outcomes than the impact of personal behavioral choices. Bad people making bad personal choices cannot be the explanation for the persistent disparities between African-Americans and Whites in their health outcomes.

Although the historical roots of these disparities may offer some explanation, they do not offer any justification. More and more groups and individuals involved in health care outcomes recognize that addressing transportation, housing, education and income offers the key to improving long-term health outcomes. Allowing people to move toward better housing with enhanced mobility represents a key to addressing health disparities. Educational opportunity improves income potential and health outcomes.

In every other part of the country, people can identify the ghetto, whether it is Black, Brown or Yellow. Everyone knows where the neighborhoods are located characterized by rent-to-own, payday loans, fast foods, liquor stores and high crime. Their boundaries are often rooted in history and predict a lifestyle and life outcomes with devastating accuracy. As many authors have pointed out, your life-expectancy depends on your zip code. Bad environmental barrels (with poor housing, failing schools, food deserts, high crime and unemployment) tend to produce bad apples. While a bad barrel may produce a remarkable apple that rises above difficult circumstances to achieve extraordinary success, that remains the exception and not the rule.

Those living in the good barrels (with good housing, good schools, high incomes, low crime and low unemployment) have neither the desire nor the expectation that they must share their good fortune. On the contrary, there are systematic barriers (often literal) erected to keep the influx of those who will bring down property values and school test scores. Again, there are notable exceptions and good barrels can produce rotten apples, but that too is the exception and not the rule. Change, sometimes halting and painful, has occurred. The New South has abandoned the Jim Crow laws and discriminatory voting rules. Yet the heritage of separate but unequal persists to this day.

Adequate public transportation, excellence in education, development of decent, low-income housing in mixed income neighborhoods and wage scales sufficient to allow more than just survival all play a role in prompting community wellbeing and health.

The Old South, poisoned by a legacy of slavery, gave way to the New South, tainted by Jim Crow. The "No South" shares its failings and opportunities with the entire nation. If we do not confront the stain of disparities and strive for equity of opportunity and the elimination of barriers, we will remain mired under the burden of Southern history.

A new dawn of opportunities that enhance health need not be out of reach. It should be the product of careful analysis, thoughtful actions and the concerted efforts of everyone to make things better.

INFECTIOUS DISEASES

AVIAN ZOONOSES: DISEASES FROM OUR FEATHERED FRIENDS

Birds enhance our environment with their songs, seed dispersal, consumption of insects, as a source of game and, of course, as family pets. Who has not owned a parakeet or parrot, or raised chickens or ducks at some time in their life? Unfortunately, birds, like many other animals, can harbor infections that can be transmitted to humans.

External parasites, both mites and lice, infect birds and can be transmitted to humans. Although we are not definitive hosts, both organisms can cause redness and itching. More troublesome are three important fungal diseases: aspergillosis, cryptococcocis and histoplasmosis. Birds become the source of human infections through droppings, which contain infectious spores. These can result in pulmonary infections, sometimes deadly in immune-compromised persons (those with low immunity).

Birds can also be infected with viruses, including West Nile Virus and Avian Influenza. Each year, we have a number of West Nile Virus cases, transmitted to humans through mosquitos that have fed on infected birds. West Nile Virus spread quickly across the United States in the late 90's and early 2000's thanks to migrations of our feathered friends. Although there are many mosquito-borne diseases (malaria, dengue, chikungunya and others), most do not co-infect birds.

Birds get their own flu, Avian Influenza, H5N1 and other strains. It kills over 50% of its human victims, but human-to-human transmission is rare and it mostly affects those with very close contact with poultry as occurs in Southeast Asia. Mutations, however, are always possible and a more transmissible bird-to-human strain could prove disastrous.

Birds also contract bacterial diseases, notably avian tuberculosis, erysipelas and psittacosis, all of which can be transmitted to humans. By far the most serious human health hazard posed by poultry in the United States is food poisoning cases caused by salmonella and campylobacter. Over 50% of poultry is contaminated with salmonella or campylobacter, resulting in periodic food related outbreaks and recalls. Eggs are also subject to contamination and should be correctly stored and cooked (and never eaten raw).

Lastly, birds carry a few protozoan infections (microscopic animals), including sarcocystis, cryptosporidium and giardia. Each year, a few of these latter two infections pop up in the United States.

In conclusion, we always need to be aware that our feathered friends can harbor diseases that we can contract. Handling pets, game and especially poultry products needs to done carefully and with adequate hand washing and reduced cross-contamination of surfaces. Yes, birds are our feathered friends; they nonetheless deserve to be treated with respect as potential sources of disease.

BIRD FLU, WHAT YA GONNA DO?

The news periodically reports cases of the dreaded "bird flu" propagating through commercial flocks in the United States. Before giving up on eating chicken or turkey, however, some information about these outbreaks of bird flu is in order. Bird flu has been around as long as human flu, probably longer. Influenza A, in one of its many variations, infects birds and mammals, including human beings. Fortunately, all strains of Influenza A do not infect all animals and, on the contrary, are often highly specific to one species or another.

Bird flu, like human strains, undergoes constant antigenic shift and drift, changing its genetic material as it circles the globe. Wild birds can be and often are infected and transmit the disease to other birds as they migrate. Wild ducks and geese, as well other avian species can pass the infection to other wild birds or to domestic flocks all over the globe.

There have been periodic epidemics of bird flu in Southeast Asia for decades, but since bird flu usually does not readily infect human beings, only a few hundred deaths occur in the worst years. These fatalities are almost always among people with a very close contact with poultry, often raising ducks or chickens in or under their homes. Although bird flu can be fatal when contracted by humans, they only rarely become infected and the human host does not easily transmit it to others humans (unlike with human strains of influenza). As mentioned, mutations are always possible which allow greatly increased bird-to-bird and human-to-human transmission as well.

The latest bird flu epidemics in the United States struck domestic flocks of chickens and turkeys. As in humans, influenza spreads quickly and easily through a domestic flock, which often numbers in the thousands. Since there is no treatment for the birds, the flocks, whether they are turkeys or chickens, must be euthanized to stop the danger of infection to other commercial flocks. The unsavory details of the process include smothering the entire flock in foam and then burying the carcasses in a pit that is then covered with dirt.

As unpleasant as this process sounds, exterminating the entire flock remains the only method of stopping accidental transmission. Workers, infected manure and contaminated equipment may also spread the virus, although the most likely source remains accidental contact with migratory birds. Mass slaughtering events have periodically affected millions of turkeys and chickens in a number of poultry producing states across the United States.

All this being said, you cannot get bird flu from eating poultry. If you happen to have an infected backyard flock, the risk of getting bird flu is almost zero unless you have unusually close contact with the birds (something much more common in Southeast Asia). Hopefully, a vaccine can be developed for commercial flocks, although the same challenges exist as with human influenza: constantly shifting virus genetics and the necessity of costly mass vaccination annually. The logistics of such a process and its cost could prove prohibitive.

Meanwhile, enjoy your chicken or turkey dinner and remember to get your human flu shot in October or whenever it becomes available. Even though the flu shot for humans does not necessarily offer complete protection from circulating human strains, it still reduces the morbidity and mortality associated with seasonal influenza.

EBOLA: JUST A PLANE FLIGHT AWAY

Ebola Viral Disease (or EVD) is one of many RNA viruses that infect humans. All viruses reproduce by high jacking the cellular machinery and making the cell produce new viruses instead of normal proteins. Ebola is one of a group of filoviruses (string-like viruses) that produce a deadly hemorrhagic fever, resulting in the death of over 50% of those infected.

Ebola is not new. Periodic epidemics have broken out in West and Central Africa since the 70's, where it is a "zoonosis" or animal-borne disease. The animal hosts include bats, non-human primates (monkeys and chimpanzees) and other creatures, some of which are consumed by humans as "bush meat." Because of this natural reservoir, total eradication of Ebola has proven impossible and periodic outbreaks, such as that in 2014 or the more recent outbreak in Central Congo in 2018, will continue to occur.

Up until now, the epidemics have had little geographic spread, often being limited to remote villages where the disease infects a few individuals and then dies out. In 2014, however, Ebola struck large urban areas in Guinea, Sierra Leone and Liberia. The latter two countries had been devastated by decades of civil wars, which left their governments and health systems in disarray.

Ebola is not airborne, although it can be transmitted on large droplets. Transmission depends on direct contact with blood, sweat, vomitus, diarrhea, semen or vaginal secretions. Once introduced, the virus invades and destroys vascular epithelial cells, resulting in massive bleeding and diarrhea. As the person becomes sicker, the viral load (the number of viruses) increases, making terminally ill patients particularly dangerous to others.

In 2014, over 5,000 people died from Ebola and over 13,000 were infected in West Africa. These unprecedented numbers posed an enormous public health challenge. In Africa, the treatment consisted of isolation and hydration, often under very primitive conditions, and over 50% of those infected died from the disease. This mortality rate has dropped closer to 30% with better supportive care. There are no specific proven medications against Ebola, but a vaccine was successfully attempted in Sierra Leone and Guinea toward the end of the 2014 epidemic. Trials are now underway with the most recent outbreak in 2018 in Central Congo.

Several notorious cases were treated in the U.S. in 2014, eight out of nine survived. Although not required, specialized bio-containment units (four of which exist around the U.S.) can accommodate up to 12 cases. In the U.S., control measures consisted of screenings of visitors from West Africa who had already been screened in their home countries. Public health workers monitored people who had been to West Africa and who were not symptomatic twice daily for 21 days. Quarantine varied depending on the symptoms and on the level of exposure in West Africa.

The first question any patients were asked in the U.S. was whether they had traveled to West Africa in the last month, specifically to Guinea, Sierra Leone or Liberia. Providers then asked if you had been in contact with anyone who had traveled in West Africa who might have Ebola. Since only symptomatic people can be infectious, you were then asked if you had fever, nausea, vomiting, diarrhea, join and muscle pains, headache or unusual fatigue. The definition of fever shifted from 101.5 degrees Fahrenheit to 100.4 and eventually became "subjective fever from baseline." If your travel history and symptoms suggested Ebola, you were isolated and the necessary laboratory work obtained.

Ebola scares the public, and rightfully so. Any disease that kills over 50% of its victims and has no specific treatment must be a source of major concern. That being said, actions should be based on science and logic, not on fear. In the end, the development of an effective vaccine (currently being used in Central Congo) and eradication of the disease among humans in West Africa will constitute our best defense in the U.S. Ebola, however, remains in the wild and will not go away, but will re-appear periodically to threaten African countries and elsewhere in this day of mass long-distance travel. Ebola remains only a plane flight away.

DENGUE AND CHIKUNGUNYA: MOSQUITO-BORNE INVADERS ON OUR BORDERS

Dengue and chikungunya are two viral diseases that are poised on our borders. Infected Aedes mosquitos, which are present throughout the Southern United States including Louisiana, transmit both diseases. Dengue is found in the Caribbean, as well as in South American, Africa and Southeast Asia. Travelers to Caribbean islands, whose numbers exceed hundreds of thousands annually, can and do become infected and bring the disease back to the U.S. Dengue has been reported in isolated indigenous (non-imported) cases in Key West, Florida and on the Texas-Mexican border.

The mosquito acquires dengue by biting an infected human and, after an incubation period of a few days, transmits the organism in its saliva when it bites another person. Once infected, there is an incubation period of about a week in humans. After that, around 25% of cases develop symptoms, with fever, severe joint and muscle pains, a diffuse rash, and spots related to platelet dysfunction (purpura).

This "febrile phase" (fever phase) is followed by a "critical phase" in around 5% of symptomatic individuals. Symptoms include abdominal pain and vomiting and may lead to hypotension and shock due to fluid shifts from the vessels to the tissues. There can be blood in the stool, pancreatitis, hepatitis and even death. Prompt recognition of this "critical phase" and aggressive fluid administration reduces mortality from 10% to only 1%.

When dengue is suspected, it can be confirmed with certain specialized lab tests (PT-PCR or DENV Non-structural protein.) Although fairly easy to diagnose, there are no specific treatments for dengue. Aspirin and similar platelet aggregation inhibitor medications should be avoided since they can worsen bleeding.

Chikungunya, another viral disease transmitted by the same mosquito, is found in Africa, Southeast Asia and also, more recently, in some Caribbean islands. Like dengue, it can cause fever, joint pain and a rash, making it difficult to differentiate from dengue in patients from susceptible areas (notably the Caribbean.) Like dengue, it can be confirmed by specialized lab tests (IgM) and has no specific treatment. The first case of a locally acquired infection in the continental U.S. was reported in Florida, where prompt and aggressive mosquito abatement and human and mosquito testing limited its spread and resulted in eradication of the focus of infection.

Prevention remains the best option, with careful avoidance of mosquito bites and effective mosquito control efforts. Unfortunately, both of these diseases could establish themselves in the Southern United States. *Aedes aegypti,* one of the mosquitos that transmit both viruses, has proven both persistent and adaptable in urban environments. The mosquito's presence, along with that of these two viral diseases, poses a constant threat across the Southern U.S.

The importation and dissemination of West Nile Virus, another mosquito-borne viral disease, serves as a constant warning that such diseases are only waiting for their opportunity to invade the United States. Fortunately, neither dengue nor chikungunya seems to infect birds, making rapid, widespread dissemination more unlikely than with West Nile virus. For more information, consult www.cdc.gov.

Another mosquito-borne disease, Zika, will be discussed in another segment.

ZIKA VIRUS: ANOTHER UNWANTED MOSQUITO-BORNE INVADER

In our days of worldwide travel, germs move with us on our meanderings. Zika virus has now grabbed the international headlines. It is a *Flavivirus*, one of several that is transmitted from human-to-human through the bite of mosquitos. In this case, as with the Dengue and chikungunya viruses, it is transmitted through the bite of *Aedes* species mosquitos, present throughout the Southern U.S. and much of the world. Zika, dengue and chikungunya could become endemic in the U.S. given the widespread presence of Aedes mosquitos, a very adaptable species.

Although Zika was previously identified in Southeast Asia and Central Africa, it made the jump to the "New World" recently, probably in 2012. Once established by means of an imported infected individual, Zika, like West Nile before it, quickly established itself and now extends throughout much of Central, South America and the Caribbean (notably Haiti and the Dominican Republic.) Although imported cases have been reported in the U.S., Zika has not established itself here yet as a widespread infection. There were a handful of human-to-human cases reported in Miami, Florida, where prompt testing and mosquito abatement eradicated the focus. There have been no human-to-human mosquito-borne infections reported there since. Direct human-to-human transmission can occur through infected sperm and appropriate contraception following infection and exposure is recommended.

As far as infections go, Zika virus is only symptomatic in about 20% of those infected and symptoms are relatively mild (rash, joint and muscle pains, headache and conjunctivitis.) Symptoms last about a week and recovery is the rule. Infection in pregnant women, however, can result in cases of microcephaly (babies born with small heads and associated neurological abnormalities.) Pediatricians in Brazil first noticed this association, and several thousand cases have now been reported. There have also been rare reported cases of *Guillain-Barré* syndrome in adults, a devastating neurological disorder, associated with Zika infection.

Zika virus is difficult to diagnosis and requires specialized blood tests that are only performed at the CDC and a few state health labs, including in Louisiana. The problem is cross-reactivity with other diseases, such as Dengue, which presents with almost identical symptoms. In fact, the non-specific symptoms of Zika virus resemble a host of other diseases, including chikungunya, rubella, measles, parovirus, adenovirus and enterovirus. The clinician must be suspicious of Zika, however, in anyone returning from the many countries where it is now endemic (see www.cdc.gov.)

Like dengue and chikungunya, Zika virus has no specific treatment. Rest, hydrations and acetaminophen (Tylenol ®) are recommended for aches and pains (rather than non-steroidal anti-inflammatory medications since these can aggravate bleeding if the disease happens to be hemorrhagic Dengue.) Pregnant women (or potentially pregnant women) should avoid travel in the infected countries listed on the CDC website. These travel restrictions posed a particular challenge during the 2016 Summer Olympics in Rio de Janeiro, Brazil. Although greatly feared, widespread infection and dissemination, however, did not become a major health problem during or after the Olympics.

As with all mosquito-borne diseases, precautions should be taken here and elsewhere to reduce exposure: limit outside activities in the early morning and evening, wear long-sleeve clothing, use DEET or other insect repellants, repair screens and reduce standing water around homes and businesses. A "simple" mosquito bite, whether in Alexandria, Louisiana, or Rio de Janeiro, Brazil, can cause a host of problems. While locally we still worry about West Nile virus, elsewhere Zika, dengue and chikungunya have established themselves firmly in many countries and are only waiting to invade the continental U.S.

INFLUENZA: MISPLACED COMPLACENCY

Most people shrug off the flu as an inevitable and annoying bother. The fact remains, however, that this worldwide recurrent scourge, depending on the severity of the strain, kills anywhere from 3,000 to 30,000 Americans each year, many of them elderly or very young. Influenza A is not just a human affliction, but infects a host of birds and mammals, and can jump from species to species with remarkable EASE. Influenza's extraordinary capacity for genetic antigenic shift and drift allows it to mutate and recombine in new and deadly combinations every year as it sweeps around the globe.

Although most Americans have only vaguely heard of the "Spanish Flu," that particular pandemic in 1918 killed around 50 million people worldwide (500,000 in the U.S. alone) and resulted in more deaths than all those killed in the First World War (around 17 million). While we now have antibiotics and intensive care units, the carnage from a 1918-like flu (with 2% mortality) would cause over a million deaths in Louisiana alone.

Flu vaccine must be altered each year to reflect the current strains of influenza. In the 2015-2016 Flu Season, the trivalent (3 component) flu vaccine contained the H1N1 (A/California), H3N2 (A/Switzerland) and B (Phuuket) viral components. These are updates from the 2014-2015 vaccines. The quadrivalent (4 element) vaccine also contains an additional B (Brisbane) viral component. Some newly approved flu vaccines include the jet injector device and Fluzone ® Intradermal Quadrivalent.

During the 2014-15, flu season the H3N2 strain underwent some significant antigenic drift (genetic changes) which reduced its effectiveness to as low as 23% protection. But mis-matching should not hinder anyone from getting vaccinated with the current preparations. Although not 100%

effective in the 2015-2016 flu season, the efficacy of flu vaccine usually approaches 60% in the best of cases.

The 2017-2018 Flu Season also held some surprises. Although the B strain appeared to be a fairly close match, the H3N2 match was again weak, with estimates of only 10% to 30% efficacy. Again, no mismatch should prevent the public from getting the flu vaccine. Some protection is always better than none.

Flu vaccination, even without a perfect match, still helps reduce the severity of the illness in those who get infected. This is especially true in high-risk groups including those over 65, those less than 2 years of age, pregnant women, the morbidly obese and the immune-compromised. Readily available in supermarkets, physicians' offices and other venues, the flu vaccine cost is usually covered by most insurance plans because of the benefits to their policyholders.

Why the largess from insurers? Simply put, the cost of the vaccines is far less than the cost of the disease. Flu causes $10 billion in absenteeism and direct medical costs every year. Sixty-two million Americans get the flu annually, and around 200,000 are hospitalized. As mentioned, anywhere between 3,000 and 30,000 will die, most of them elderly, but some young children and some chronically ill persons of any age as well. This proved true in the 2017-2018 epidemic.

While many children (56%) and older Americans (66%) get vaccinated, only 35% of young adults bother to do so. Healthy People 2020 goals are to achieve 80% vaccination rates in children, 70% in young adults, and 90% of all senior citizens and healthcare workers. The latter group is of particular interest because, left to their own devices, only about 67% of healthcare workers choose to be vaccinated. This jumps to over 90% when flu vaccination is mandated by healthcare employer policy that can impose mask wearing, suspensions or dismissal of employees.

Although other diseases such as Legionnaire's or Ebola may capture the headlines from time to time, it is important to remember our wily viral enemy, influenza, and get vaccinated whether it is mandated or not. The cost of vaccination is minimal, but the cost of influenza may be as high as death.

LEGIONNAIRES' DISEASE: ANOTHER UBIQUITOUS HAZARD

Periodic outbreaks of Legionnaires' disease bring this ubiquitous infection back into public prominence from time to time. Present in water, notably in cooling towers, humidifiers, spas, misters and even showerheads, Legionnaires' disease occurs in isolated cases or multiple-case outbreaks, including occasional hospital-acquired infections. The disease is not transmitted from person-to-person, but only occurs with environmental exposure (usually as contaminated inhaled mist).

The agent is a Gram-negative bacterium, *Legionella pneumophilia*, which occurs worldwide. It achieved fame and its name when a number of American Legionnaires became ill following a convention in 1976. Since then, it causes anywhere from 8,000 to 18,000 cases every year. Besides the severe pneumonia associated with Legionella, it can also cause a mild, non-pulmonary disease called Pontiac Fever.

Most cases of Legionnaires' disease begin with a flu-like syndrome of generalized aches and pains, followed by fever, cough, diarrhea and abdominal pains. A chest x-ray shows patchy infiltrates and blood (and/or urine) tests confirm the diagnosis. While Pontiac fever is self-limiting and does not require antibiotics, full blown Legionnaires' disease can result in a 50% death rate and requires prompt treatment with specific antibiotics (fluoroquinolones or doxycycline for 2-3 weeks).

As in the case of many infectious diseases, the severity of the case is often related to the age and general condition of the infected individual, with the elderly (over 50), immune suppressed, smokers, diabetics, and those with renal or hepatic failure having the highest risk of death. The male to female ration is 2.5:1 and the disease is rare in people under 20 years of age.

From a physician's standpoint, Legionnaires' disease should be considered in someone presenting with a severe pneumonia, often elderly, with diabetes, cancer, COPD and kidney or liver failure, with a recent history of travel (within two weeks, especially if spa use was reported), failure of other antibiotic treatments, or exposure to Legionella in the hospital setting. The disease, once diagnosed, must be reported to the Office of Public Health. Additional cases will be sought in business and household contacts or in hospital personnel when the case is identified in a healthcare institution.

If the source of Legionella is in a cooling tower, it must be drained and then cleaned regularly to remove plaque and sediment. Biocides (special cleaning solutions) should be used to reduce growth of slime (biofilm)-producing organisms that can harbor Legionella. Hot water systems should be maintained at 122 degrees Fahrenheit, and tap water should not be used in respiratory therapy aerosol machines.

Now, after hearing all the scary information about Legionnaires' disease, enjoy the trip you have planned and take advantage of the gorgeous spa. But if you come down with a flu-like syndrome, fever and cough two weeks later, please let your doctor know.

LISTERIA: DEADLY FOOD POISONING FOR YOUNG AND OLD

Food poisoning is common, affecting over 48 million Americans each year. While food poisoning can be caused by a number of organisms, *Listeria monocytogenes* is one that can cause death. Around 1,600 people a year are sickened by Listeria each year and it is the third leading cause of death from food poisoning.

While the absolute number of cases appears small, the vast majority (90%) of victims are pregnant women, their fetuses and newborns, the elderly and people with compromised immune systems. The latter group includes people with chronic diseases and those taking medications that affect their immune response (i.e. steroids, immuno-biologicals and anti-cancer drugs.)

Listeria often occurs in prepared meats (i.e. hotdogs), sprouts, soft cheeses, deli meats, raw milk and smoked salmon. More rarely, it contaminates fruits (cantaloupe) or vegetables (celery). Unlike many germs, listeria resists cold and can grow in refrigerated foods. It can also contaminate equipment and the food prepared using it.

Once infection occurs, listeria can be transmitted via the blood to a fetus and result in stillbirths or newborn deaths. In other victims, especially the elderly, it can be carried in the bloodstream to the brain and cause fatal meningitis.

While it is almost impossible to recognize infected foods, prompt detection and removal of the contaminated products is key to limiting outbreaks. Techniques of serotyping permit the identification of specific serotypes that cause over 95% of human illness. While it took 31 days to identify an outbreak associated with soft cheese in 1985, it took only 7 days to identify an outbreak associated with cantaloupe in 2011. Fortunately, cases have decreased from 8/1,000,000 people in 1950 to only around 2/1,000,000 in 2015.

Besides prompt recognitions, strict adherence to USDA guidelines for the preparation of ready-to-eat meat and poultry products is helpful. Outbreak recognition using disease surveillance specialists working with state (or national) Infectious Disease-Epidemiology personnel proves especially effective.

On an individual level, consumers can heat hot dogs completely, never drink raw milk, avoid *queso fresco* (Mexican soft cheese), refrigerate leftovers at 40 degree F or lower within two hours of use and consume within four days. Consumers can also avoid cross contamination between meat products and other foods by cleaning countertops and cutting boards (preferably not wood) thoroughly.

MUMPS (EPIDEMIC PAROTITIS): ALMOST GONE, BUT NOT ENTIRELY

Mumps, also called Epidemic Parotitis, is caused by a paramyxovirus with a predilection for the salivary glands. Prior to the initiation of mumps vaccination in 1967, there were over 186,000 cases reported each year. After that, the numbers dropped from several thousand to several hundred a year at most.

Mumps enters the body through saliva or droplets entering the nose or mouth. After a 14 to 24 day incubation period, some people develop painful swelling of the parotid glands (large salivary glands near the back of the jaw) accompanied by headache, fever, and malaise. This only occurs in 30 to 65% of infected individuals, while another 15 to 27% have no symptoms at all. Some people may develop only cold-like symptoms, with mild fever and loss of appetite.

In those with fever, it usually subsides after a few days as does the parotid swelling. In post-pubescent individuals, the virus can also attack the testicles (or ovaries), pancreas and the brain causing orchitis in males, pancreatitis and meningitis respectively. Long-term consequences are rare, but some males may develop testicular atrophy (which does not effect fertility).

Pancreatitis may occur a week after infection and will subside a week later without residual problems. Meningitis, while painful and sometimes associated with seizures or even coma, also usually resolves without long term harm. Deafness in one ear or both occurs rarely (1/20,000 reported cases).

With almost complete vaccination among children at 12 months and 5 years of age (in the combined MMR or Measles-Mumps-Rubella vaccine), it might be surprising that any cases of mumps occur at all. Unfortunately, there are always a few unvaccinated adults and children and the vaccine is only 88% effective at best in those having received the vaccine. This means that outbreaks among closely clustered populations can and do occur, notably on college campuses.

While most years there are only a few hundred cases, as mentioned above, in 2006 there were around 6,500 cases. There was another spike in 2016 to 5,800 and there were already over 3,000 cases in 2017, most of them in Arkansas. Louisiana also reported 63 cases (through June, 2017), most of them among LSU students and a few other sporadic cases elsewhere. Almost 1,500 students received MMR vaccinations in Louisiana following this outbreak.

Repeat vaccination among previously vaccinated adults is not generally recommended with the exception of close contacts to known documented cases (such as the university students in Louisiana). Documented cases are those that have been confirmed by laboratory testing (a buccal swab for RT-PCR). Infected individuals should be isolated because they are infectious three days prior to symptoms and five days after developing symptoms.

There is no treatment for mumps besides supportive care. A soft, acid-free diet reduces painful chewing. Patients with vomiting may require IV fluids. Men with orchitis (painful swelling of the testicle) benefit from ice packs and scrotal support.

Despite warnings from a tenacious group of ill-informed adults who oppose vaccinations, the MMR (measles-mumps-rubella) vaccine is safe and effective. All children should be vaccinated at 12 months and again at 5 years. Side effects from vaccination may include a slight fever (10%) and rash (5%). The only people who should not be vaccinated are those who are allergic to the vaccine and pregnant women or severely immuno-compromised individuals (since it is a live virus vaccine). The benefits of vaccination hugely outweigh any minor inconveniences. The near eradication of mumps, measles and rubella, with their horrific complications, has been one of the triumphs of modern medicine and public health.

RODENTS, OUR DEADLY
LITTLE NEIGHBORS

When people think of rodents, especially rats and mice, they usually consider them as more or less harmless household pests. In fact, rodents cause anywhere from 500,000 to a million dollars or more of crop damage and food contamination every year. They also cause a high percentage of house fires by gnawing through electrical wires. Still worse, they can cause a number of serious human diseases.

Native U.S. rodents include woodchucks, groundhogs, squirrels and chipmunks. All can carry plague, tularemia and tick borne typhus. But by far the most common rodent vectors are the "imported species," which includes the Norway rat, roof rat and house mouse, all originating in Asia. Over 14,000 rodent bites occur annually, at a rate of about 10/100,000 population, and several hundred rodent-borne illnesses are treated each year.

How do rats spread disease? It depends on the disease, but they can spread illness through bites, fecal and urine contamination of food or water, or through intermediaries such as fleas, ticks or mites. One rat produces a pound of urine and 50 fecal pellets a day, plenty for abundant contamination.

So what are the specific rodent-related diseases? First, Rat Bite Fever (or Haverhill Fever) is a febrile illness caused by *Streptobacillus villiformis*, a bacterium. It can be acquired through bites or scratches or through urine or fecal contamination. From 30-50% of the rodent population may be infected. Sewage workers, hunters, veterinarians, pet owners and nature travelers can all become infected. Death can occur in 5% of cases, especially in those over 65 years of age.

Murine typhus (a rickettsial disease) occurs in three forms: endemic, scrub or murine. Infected fleas or lice transmit typhus after biting an infected rodent, usually a flying squirrel. A rare disease (less than 100 cases per year) in our times, it caused devastation in the trenches in World War I. Now, if correctly diagnosed, it can be treated with tetracycline or chloramphenicol.

Eosinophilic meningitis (a strongyloid infection) and lymphocytic choriomeningitis (a virus), both attack the central nervous system. The latter disease is found in around 5% of house mice. Eosinophilic meningitis is acquired by accidently eating vegetables infested with contaminated snails and slugs that have eaten infected rat feces or urine. Both cause serious headaches and can be rapidly fatal in rare cases (around 1% for cases of lymphocytic choriomeningitis.)

Native rodents (ground squirrel and chipmunks among them) spread Hantavirus Pulmonary Syndrome, a serious, sometime fatal lung disease. Infected fecal matter is found in the walls of rustic housing and inhaled by the residents. It is "species specific" (different viruses in different rodent species) and although rare (only 45 cases since 2006), it results in a 30% mortality rate.

Other rodent-related diseases include hemorrhagic fever with renal syndrome, rickettsialpox (occurring in large Eastern U.S. cities) and better-known illnesses such as plague, trichinosis and toxoplasmosis. Plague occurs sporadically around the world, especially in rural areas. Domestic and feral hogs eat rats infected with trichinosis and become the leading cause of that disease in human who consume inadequately cooked pork. Toxoplasmosis also occurs in cats (acquired through contact with infected rodents) and they transmit the spores in their feces. Pregnant women should never clean kitty litter boxes for that reason. Toxoplasmosis can be devastating to the developing fetus.

In short, rats and mice and other rodents cause destruction and spread disease. Trap and remove mice and rats if they invade your home. Be sure to secure your home by sealing cracks, crevices and holes and make sure all food products in your home are safely stored. Always handle rodents (including pet rats and mice) with gloves. The very young and very old are always more susceptible to rodent-borne diseases and children less than 6 years old should not handle rodents (or reptiles) at all.

So whether the rodents are native or imported, wild or pets, they should all be recognized as potential sources of disease and treated as such.

SEPSIS: SILENT KILLER

Sepsis is when germs, from any number of potential sources, enter the bloodstream and are disseminated around the body, affecting multiple organs. People of all ages may be affected, but we will concentrate on adults, particularly the elderly. As with many medical conditions, the consequences can be deadly, especially for the very old and very young.

A large study, published in CDC's Morbidity and Mortality Weekly Report (August 23, 2016) helped put a spotlight on the epidemiology of sepsis from four large acute care hospitals in New York. Their results, based on 246 adult cases, revealed that 26% of these patients died (72% of them aged 65 or older). Most of the adult patients with sepsis (97%) had some significant underlying medical condition: diabetes mellitus (35%), cardiovascular disease (32%), chronic kidney disease (23%) and/or COPD (Chronic Obstructive Pulmonary Disease) (20%).

The infectious diseases that triggered sepsis in this largely pre-disposed populations were pneumonia (35%), urinary tract infections (25%), gastrointestinal infections (11%) and skin infections (11%). The incriminated germs were mostly Staphylococcus, E. coli and Streptococcus, as well as some others. Most of these cases were actually acquired prior to hospitalizations (58%) while fewer (42%) were acquired in the hospital setting.

Besides resulting in death (25%) and morbidity that prolongs hospital stays and requires long-term care post-hospitalizations, sepsis costs an estimated $23.7 billion a year in cumulative medical expenses. This terrible medical problem is, to some extent, avoidable. Since pneumonias account for a large number of cases, vaccination against influenza and pneumococcus can reduce susceptibility. Unfortunately, in this study, which reflects the general U.S. population, only 44% of the adults had received their pneumococcal vaccine and only 35% were vaccinated against influenza. The goal is, of course, complete vaccination, especially in the elderly.

Awareness of hospital-acquired infections has increased along with increased measures of hand hygiene, use of appropriate protective equipment and strict monitoring of the rates of Central Line-associated Bloodstream Infections (CLABSIs). Healthcare professions and family members are also encouraged to recognize the early symptoms of sepsis, which are sometimes subtle and confusing, especially in the elderly. Signs and symptoms often include fever, generalized pain, clammy skin, shortness of breath, tachycardia (fast heart rate) and confusion.

Rapid recognition and treatment can improve outcomes. Prevention of infections through vaccinations and hand washing, education of family members and healthcare providers, rapid treatment and prompt reassessment of appropriate therapy are all keys to a successful outcome. That being said, sepsis still remains a high morbidity and mortality condition that threatens all ages, especially the elderly.

Shannon A. Novosad et al. Epidemiology of Sepsis: Prevalence of Health Care Factors and Opportunities for Prevention. MMWR. Early Release/Vol. 65. August, 2016.

SEXUALLY TRANSMITTED DISEASES: UPDATE FOR LOUISIANA AND CENLA

There are many sexually transmitted diseases, but those that are tracked and quantified in Louisiana and nationally include gonorrhea, chlamydia and primary and secondary syphilis. Although HIV/AIDS is also transmitted sexually, it is often tracked separately.

Louisiana has the dubious honor of ranking in the top 4 states in the U.S. with respect to sexually transmitted disease (STD) rates that vary only slightly from year to year. In 2017, Louisiana ranked #1 for primary, secondary and congenital syphilis and #2 for gonorrhea and chlamydia and #3 for HIV/AIDS. These extraordinary statistics translate into significant morbidity and economic loss.

CENLA has its share of cases, but does not rank at the top of Louisiana public health regions with respect to any of these diseases. Out of the nine Louisiana public health regions, CENLA ranked 5/9 for gonorrhea, 6/9 for chlamydia and 7/9 for syphilis. Although we are doing better than many other parts of Louisiana, we still have tremendous room for improvement when compared with national statistics. And who wants to be in the top five states, year after year for decades?

There are some significant demographic differences with respect to STDs both in the nation, the state and our region. In our region, cases for both gonorrhea and chlamydia are more commonly diagnosed in women, 64% and 73% respectively (not unlike state or national statistics). Some of this relates to "sampling error" since sexually active women are systematically checked for STDs in annual gynecological exams (at least in the context of the health units) and men only seek assistance when symptomatic. With syphilis, on the contrary, over 85% of those diagnosed regionally are men (similar to state and national figures), which is skewed by the high incidence of syphilis cases in the population of men having sex with men.

Not only are there disparities with sex, but also with ethnicity. For reasons probably related to low income and lower educational attainment rather than race, African-Americans are disproportionately represented in all STDs (and HIV/AIDS) regionally, with 79% of cases of gonorrhea, 60% of chlamydia cases and 69% of those with primary and secondary syphilis. The same holds true with HIV/AIDS, with about 75% of cases in African Americans both regionally and in the state as a whole. Again, there may be some "sampling error" because STD's are systematically checked in sexually active women in certain age groups in the health units, but not necessarily in the private sector where more patients with non-Medicaid insurance are seen.

With both gonorrhea and chlamydia, the majority of cases in CENLA (69% and 74% respectively) occur in the 15 to 24 year old range, hardly a surprise in this high-risk, sexually active age group. Syphilis, on the contrary, occurs more often in older adults, with 62% of cases in the 25 to 44 year old group, with most of these cases in men who have sex with men (MSM) and an over representation of African-Americans.

The high rates of STDs (and HIV/AIDs) in our region and in the state should underline the importance of responsible sexual choices. The only sure method for prevention is, of course, abstinence, which is laudable, but not necessarily realistic. While they do not absolutely prevent STDs, the practice of "safe sex" with the use of condoms greatly reduces the risk of contracting any sexually transmitted disease, including HIV.

Since young people are the primary recipients and transmitters of STDs, they should receive adequate education about the risks and consequences of infection in a clear, dispassionate and scientifically accurate manner, something that is not often the case. While this ideally should come from the family, parents may lack the knowledge, skill or the will to correctly transmit this information. In addition, many people are unaware that they have a STD or HIV (around 25% of cases) because they are both often asymptomatic. So appropriate testing, at least annually in some cases, and contact tracking by the Office of Public Health for syphilis and HIV can help reduce the risk of transmission in the general population.

Adolescents, by their neurobiological makeup, are saturated with hormones and yet lack complete development of the frontal lobe where reason and impulse control originate. Their impulsive decision-making and lack of self control provides a perfect storm for high-risk behavior, whether it is drug or alcohol use, driving without a seatbelt, or engaging in unprotected sex. Proper education (from whatever reliable source), avoidance of high-risk environments and role-playing for adolescents to develop automatic healthy behaviors can offer hope for improving our dreadful state and regional STD statistics.

Since 2017, Regional STD/HIV Reduction Taskforces have been established around Louisiana in hopes of engaging a broad range of providers and stakeholders. Such a collaborative approach may at least allow us to make some progress in reducing STD rates in Louisiana. Let's try and be in the top five of states for something besides STDs.

SYPHILIS STRIKES BACK!

Louisiana ranks #1 among U.S. states for its rates of primary and secondary syphilis and congenital syphilis. Despite aggressive public health campaigns and follow-ups among contacts by trained public health agents, this insidious sexually transmitted disease has not been eliminated. In fact, new cases are increasing. Rates of syphilis are particularly high among African-Americans, notably in the population of men who have sex with men (MSM). Heterosexuals, homosexuals and bisexuals of all races, of course, can and do contract syphilis since it strikes indiscriminately.

Although its actual origins are still debated, syphilis has been with us for a long time. Some believe Christopher Columbus's sailors contracted syphilis from the Arawak Indians in the Caribbean and brought it back to Europe in the early 1500s. It then spread rapidly around the Old World and was known as the "Spanish Disease," or the "French Disease" or the "Italian Disease" depending on the country.

The infectious agent is a spirochete (*Treponema pallidum*), a microscopic snake-like creature that requires special microscopic techniques to directly visualize it (dark field exam). Until the development of penicillin, there was no effective treatment. With the advent of penicillin, to which the spirochete is still sensitive, an effective treatment became available and huge strides were made toward eliminating the disease.

After World War II, the rates of syphilis plummeted and some hoped it would disappear entirely. That, however, has not proven to be the case. Syphilis rates never reached zero and have steadily increased over the last few decades.

Why should this be true? In fact, syphilis, one of many sexually transmitted diseases, has a very complex clinical presentation. Once inoculated through sexual contact, the newly infected individual develops primary syphilis, which manifests itself as a painless ulcer (or chancre) with a hard base. This lesion, teeming with spirochetes, occurs at the point of contact, which may be on the vagina, penis, anus or even the lip. This painless ulcer, often unapparent in women, may induce the patient to apply local creams or lotions or do nothing at all. If they are wise enough to consult a medical provider, syphilis may be confirmed with a blood test and the patient will be treated with 2.4 million units of intramuscular benzathine penicillin (a 1.2 million unit shot in each buttocks) as a one time treatment and cure.

If the infected person does not seek treatment, the lesion (or chancre) clears up by itself, while the individual remains infectious to others. After several weeks on months, however, the untreated syphilis (now secondary syphilis) manifests itself as a disseminated rash, sometimes associated with patchy hair loss or fleshy lesions on the genitals or anus (called *condyloma accuminata*.) The highly variable rash, which does not itch or bleed, can be more prominent on the hands and feet. Once again, if diagnosed correctly (which is not always the case) with appropriate blood tests, it can be successfully treated with weekly shots of penicillin for three weeks and the patient is cured. Unfortunately, even if untreated, the rash still goes away while the person remains infectious to sexual contacts.

If the patient passes through primary and secondary syphilis without being treated, the spirochetes remain in them and the person eventually develops tertiary syphilis after many years. This causes major neurological problems, including loss of balance, blindness and dementia among other manifestations. This stage, too, can be treated successfully, but with a more complicated regimen of intravenous penicillin delivered every 4 hours for 10-14 days.

Sadly, syphilis can also be passed from an infected pregnant mother to her fetus. Congenital syphilis, as it is called, causes major developmental abnormalities including deformed teeth, neurological issues (including visual loss), and other devastating structural problems. First and third trimester syphilis testing should allow diagnosis and prompt, effective treatment of the mother, even in cases of re-infection during pregnancy.

As mentioned, because of its complex clinical manifestations, especially with primary and secondary syphilis, symptoms will disappear without treatment while the individual remains infectious to their sexual contacts. Much like HIV, around 25% of those infected with syphilis are not aware they have the disease. Systematic condom use reduces, but does not eliminate risk entirely.

In an effort to reduce our shockingly high rates of syphilis, the Office of Public Health and its HIV/STD Program have initiated a statewide campaign to increase awareness, testing and treatment of syphilis (and other STDs). STD/HIV Reduction Task Forces, comprised of medical providers and other community partners have been established in each OPH region to tackle the syphilis epidemic.

There is no reason that Louisiana must be on the top of the syphilis (and other STDs) list. Like so many of our health problems, syphilis shows notable racial disparities that require community recognition and mobilization. This awareness must be followed by the political will to allocate the necessary resources to strike back at syphilis in hope of eliminating this insidious enemy.

TUBERCULOSIS: A PERSISTENT MENACE TO HEALTH

For many people, tuberculosis (TB) seems like a disease of the distant past, yet it remains a constant threat to public health both in the United States and abroad. Worldwide, one third of people are infected with TB and 9.6 million people have become sick with the disease, which caused 1.5 million deaths, many in people co-infected with HIV.

While TB (caused by *Mycobacterium tuberculosis*) does not ravage the United States, there were still 9,421 cases in 2014. This is a far cry from the over 25,000 cases reported in 1992. In fact, there has been a steady decline in the number of cases over the last two decades.

Who gets TB in the United States today? While TB can strike anyone, 85% of the cases occur in adults over 25 years of age. More men become infected than woman at all ages, and Asians (32%), Hispanics (29%) and Blacks (21%) represent over 80% of cases. There is a clear distinction between U.S. born and foreign-born cases with the percentage of foreign-born cases surpassing U.S. born cases since 2001 and steadily increasing since then. While all TB cases are dropping, foreign-born cases now represent 66% of new cases, with 46% being Asian, 34% Hispanic and 13% Black. White foreign-born cases represent only 4% of the total number of cases.

U.S. born cases also had socioeconomic racial disparities with 37% in Blacks, 30% White, 21% Hispanic and only 3% in Asian Americans. Blacks continue to have a high number of cases with respect to their population numbers (a disparity that also occurs in HIV/AIDS). The co-existence of the two diseases (TB and HIV) reflects the increased TB infections in immune compromised HIV subjects. This association is particularly devastating in Sub-Saharan Africa where HIV-TB co-infection results in significantly increased mortality and reduction in life expectancies.

TB, which is transmitted by air, mostly affects the lungs, although it can occur in many other organs. For those with TB infection, the most common symptoms are fever, night sweats, cough (sometimes with bloody sputum), weight loss and fatigue. These symptoms may be associated with an abnormal chest X-ray, which may show cavitary lesions or other signs of inflammation.

While the formal diagnosis depends on identifying TB organisms in sputum, there are at least two screening tests that can be performed. The first is the TST or Tuberculin Skin Test in which PPD (Purified Protein Derivative), a tuberculin antigen, is injected in the skin and the diameter of the response is measured 48 to 72 hours later. Many foreign citizens receive the BCG vaccine for TB in their native countries that may make the skin test falsely positive indefinitely without corresponding latent TB infection.

The other TB tests are blood tests (T-Spot® and Quantiferon Tb Gold®), sophisticated measurements of interferon-gamma from lymphocytes exposed to TB antigens. These are blood tests which, when negative, can rule out a false-positive skin test. Health care providers are often tested annually with either the skin test or blood test, depending on the institution.

Once diagnosed, the TB patient, whether with latent TB or an active infection, is referred to the Office of Public Health where treatment is initiated. There are several treatment options for active TB, some shorter than other, and some that require Directly Observed Therapy (or DOT). The TB organism is sometimes resistant to one or another treatment medication, which requires the use of more complex medical regimens. "Multidrug Resistant Tuberculosis" (MDR TB) and "Extensively Drug Resistant TB" (XDR TB) pose particular challenges and require expert management by specialists. Without treatment, the mortality and contagion related to resistant TB can be significant.

There are also sophisticated genetic tests for the TB organism that can help differentiate between isolated and clustered cases. Such tests help specialized disease intervention specialists in public health to track down and identify contacts to known TB cases so that treatment, if needed, can be initiated.

There are those who have no symptoms and no abnormalities on the chest X-ray, but who are positive for either the T-Spot® or Quantiferon Tb Gold®. These individuals are considered to have "latent TB infection" or (LTBI). At some time in their lives, they were exposed to and retained *Mycobacterium tuberculosis* that did not cause an infection. TB could become activated in these individuals if they develop reduced immunity if given certain medications (i.e. steroids, immune-biologicals, and some cancer treatments).

These patients with "latent tuberculosis" must be treated to eliminate the possibility of TB activation at some future date. Such individuals are not sick or infectious, but still must be treated with either a six-month course or a shorter directly observed course. Due to regular TB testing, many cases of Latent TB (LTBI) are identified in health care personnel, particularly those who are foreign born. Treatments are usually well tolerated, but side effects are more likely in patients over 35 years of age.

In short, TB is still among us. It still poses a significant danger and occurs disproportionately among minority U.S. born citizens as well as in foreign-born citizens. We must still remain vigilant, especially in the medical setting, where one infected individual can wreak havoc among hospitalized patients and medical care workers alike.

WEST NILE: ANOTHER YEAR

In Louisiana, as of November 2017 (usually the end of the West Nile season), we had 40 cases of human West Nile: 36 neuroinvasive, eight febrile cases and six asymptomatic (detected through blood donations) cases, with three reported deaths. Louisiana's peak year for West Nile infections occurred in 2002 (with 204 cases of neuroinvasive disease and 124 cases of febrile disease). Afterwards, there was a steady annual decline in cases until 2012 when a huge surge occurred in both neuroinvasive (160 cases) and febrile (131 cases) disease. The following four years since 2012 have shown a dramatic reduction in reported West Nile illness with only 37 neuroinvasive cases in 2016.

The disease usually peaks in the late summer and early fall, and drops off with the cold of winter. Complacency, however, is not warranted. Neuroinvasive disease may be fatal and we have already had three such deadly cases in Louisiana as of September 2017.

Mosquitos, as most people know, transmit West Nile. Because birds are a reservoir of West Nile Virus, infected birds provide a constant source of potential human infections via mosquitos biting birds and then humans. What is less generally known is that 90% of West Nile cases are asymptomatic (no symptoms at all), only around 9% of cases have fever and an unfortunate 1%, mostly senior citizens, will develop possibly fatal neuroinvasive disease.

Why is there an apparent 10-year cycle of increased West Nile Virus cases? No one knows for sure. It might have to do with changing bird populations or the infection of groups of birds that have not previously been exposed or infected.

Besides West Nile, our indigenous mosquitos, notably *Aedes aegypti* and *Aedes albopictus*, also transmit Eastern and Western Equine and St.

Louis encephalitis, all of which are present in Louisiana, where they mostly infect horses. The same mosquitos are also capable of transmitting malaria, yellow fever, dengue, chikungunya fever and Zika, none of which are present in Louisiana except as imported cases. Mosquitos also transmit heartworm, which does not infect humans, but causes illness in dogs and cats.

All of us, especially the elderly who are more susceptible to serious cases, need to be very aware of mosquito borne illnesses, including West Nile Fever. More than just a nuisance, mosquitos can transmit a host of potentially fatal illnesses both here in Louisiana, and especially when travelling abroad (notably in South American and the Caribbean islands for dengue, chikungunya and Zika.) Remember to wear long sleeve clothing and apply mosquito repellant (usually DEET containing.) Avoid outdoor exposure in the early morning and evening (dawn and dusk) when mosquitos are most likely to feed. Remove standing water around the home and make sure screens are in good repair. Protect your pets from prolonged outdoor exposure as well, since they, too, can suffer from mosquito borne illness, heartworm.

PEDIATRICS

CHILD ABUSE AND NEGLECT: AN ONGOING TRAGEDY

Child "maltreatment," as it is called, remains a serious problem in the United States and in Louisiana. There are 3.4 million referrals to child protective services in the U.S. each year of which over 700,000 (or 9.2/1,000) are confirmed cases of "maltreatment." Most of the victims (78%) were neglected, 9% sexual abused and 11% suffered other forms of maltreatment (i.e. emotional abuse, lack of supervision, parental substance abuse or other.)

Unreported cases dwarf reported ones and child protective services estimates that 25% of all children are maltreated in some way at some time during their childhood. This results in over 1,600 child deaths a year (in 2015), most of these cases being children under the age of 6 years old (37%). More boys die than girls (2.5 vs. 1.9/100,000) and more African-American children than whites (4.7 vs. 1.6/100,000). The economic cost is also staggering, an estimated $124 billion dollar in the U.S. and over $2.7 million in Central Louisiana ($1.1 million in Rapides Parish alone.)

Who are the perpetrators of these crimes? Around 90% of abusers are related to the victims in some way. Around 40% are parents, and around 51% are other relatives (with some being unmarried parents of the victim). Most of the perpetrators are between 18 and 44 years of age (77%), while 13% are 13 to 17 years old and 10% are under 13 years of age. Most abusers are female (54%).

Risk factors vary for the perpetrators (mostly parents) and children. Parental risk factors include depression, domestic violence or history of childhood victimization, substance abuse, separation or divorce, single parent households, social isolation, poverty, unemployment and high-risk neighborhoods. Child Risk factors include prematurity (low birth weights), disability (physical or mental), young age and behavioral issues (sometimes a result of persistent neglect.)

Sadly, only 25% of children report abuse or neglect when it occurs and only another 25% will report it prior to their 18th birthday. That means 50% will never disclose their victimization prior to adulthood, and among those non-reporters, some will continue the cycle of abuse with their own children. Reporting cases by those in contact with victims becomes critical to stopping this destructive cycle.

There are a host of mandated reporters including: health providers (including mental health), social workers, clergy, child care providers, teachers, law enforcement, mediators, CASA personnel, youth activity providers, film processors and ALL adults who have witnessed sexual abuse of a child. Cases should be reported immediately, with the name, address, sex and race of the child and what you have witnessed. Reporters are not investigators. Reports should be made at 1-855-4LA-KIDS (1-855-452-5437) 24 hours a day/7 days a week or call 911.

The assessment of the situation includes an evaluation of the extent of danger (present or impending), the extent of the maltreatment, circumstances, functional capacity of the child and caregiver, parental practices (including discipline). The functional level of the care giver (intoxication, violence, hostility to intervention and level of control) and child (anxiety, independence, mental and physical state) should also be determined.

Failure to report cases of child sexual abuse by any mandated reporter can result in a $10,000 fine, 5 years in prison (possibly with hard labor) and felony charges. Worse yet, there is a good chance that victimization will continue, with increasing physical and psychological consequences, possibly resulting in death. Reporters, once they have filed a report, need not inform their supervisors, who cannot prevent reporting under any circumstances. Your name, as a reporter, cannot be released. Should another episode of abuse be witnessed, re-reporting is necessary.

Child maltreatment is pervasive and destructive. Addressing social determinants (income, educational level and social status), as in most issues related to mental and physical health, plays a critical role in prevention and treatment. The psychological scars of victimization last a lifetime and predispose victims to a cycle of repeated abuse. Let's stop the harm now and make Louisiana a better and safer place for its most vulnerable citizens.

Report child maltreatment (abuse and neglect) to 1-855-452-5437 or 911. Make the call, it's the law!

HUMAN PAPILLOMA VIRUS: PREVENTABLE WITH ADOLESCENT VACCINATION

Human Papilloma Virus (HPV) is a sexually transmitted disease that infects both women and men. It causes unsightly genital warts as well as cervical cancer in women and head and neck cancers in both sexes. When it was first introduced, the HPV vaccination raised hopes of eliminating cervical cancer, which kills around 10,000 women a year. Unfortunately, inconsistent use has prevented this vaccine from fulfilling its promise.

Although HPV vaccine can be given to children as young as 9, most girls (or boys) receive the first of three shots at 11 years of age, with the goal of completing the series prior to them becoming sexually active. If the series is given prior to age 15, only two shots are required. Achieving full vaccination, however, has proven to be frustrating both nationwide and in Louisiana.

While the target goal of Healthy People 2020 remains 80% vaccination among both girls and boys, the reality is not as cheerful. In girls 13-17, only 60% of Louisiana girls take at least one dose and only 42% complete the suggested 3 doses. Among boys, the results are even more dismal, with only 27% getting at least one shot and a meager 13% completing all three. National statistics are actually a bit worse, with only 57% of girls 13-17 getting one shot and only 38% completing the 3-shot series. Nationally, somewhat more boys get the first shot (35% vs. 27%), while about the same low number (around 14%) actually compete all three. Reducing the number of shots to only two in younger adolescents (less than 15) may improve statistics somewhat, but will not be a panacea.

In any case, the low HPV vaccination rates are a far cry from the hoped for goals. In contrast, for TDaP (Tetanus-Diphtheria and Pertussis) and Meningitis A, the Louisiana rates are a respectable 88% and 93% respectively among young people. The explanation for the difference in compliance is related to the mandatory nature of these two vaccines for enrollment in 6th grade for 11 year olds vs. the "recommended but not required" status for HPV vaccination.

Clearly, a substantial disconnect remains between what we can do with HPV vaccination and what actually is being accomplished. A vaccine that prevents genital warts and cervical (and throat) cancers from HPV should be a no-brainer among providers and the general public. Yet there remains a confused opposition, born of ignorance or misinformation, among the general public against what should be a mandatory vaccination for pre-adolescent children. Facts, not fear, should be the guiding principle in health-related matters.

Get your children (or grandchildren) vaccinated for HPV. Remember, if they complete the series by age 15, only 2 shots are required. After age 15, three shots will be needed. Completing the HPV series in order to eliminate cervical cancer in women and genital warts in both sexes should be the norm, not the exception.

INFANT DEATHS AND LOUISIANA

Many factors contribute to fetal and infant deaths. As with most unfavorable health outcomes, three factors seem to contribute: poverty, low educational level and low social status (the SES or "socioeconomic factors.") In Louisiana, as in other states, these factors are inextricably tied with race, either African-American or Hispanic, resulting in disparities in health outcomes so discouraging to Southern states.

The fact remains that more infants die in Louisiana than in almost any other state. Louisiana is 49/50 (10.9% of births) for low birth weights, 48/50 (8.2/1000 live births) for infant mortality, 49/50 (15.6% of births) for preterm births and 45/50 (8.2/1,000 live births) for teenage births. Such grim statistics, always worse in those with low socio-economic status, are even unequally distributed throughout Louisiana. The Central and Northern Mississippi River parishes suffer worse outcomes, including those for low birth weights, than other parts of Louisiana. In Central Louisiana, our highest rates for small babies, often premature and with worse outcomes are Avoyelles (11.4%), Catahoula (12.9%) and Concordia (14.8%). Despite these three parishes, CENLA's infant mortality rate for 2014-2016 remains the lowest in the state, although not lower than the national average.

The Fetal-Infant Mortality Review and Child Death Review, as well as the associated Community Action and Advisory Team, meet on successive months in each Public Health Region in the state to examine infant deaths and explore and enhance programs to reduce them. In CENLA, all sudden and unexpected infant death cases are reviewed, with input from medical and non-medical personnel with expertise in different fields. Over 75 Sudden Unexplained Infant Deaths (SUIDS) occur in Louisiana each year and represent around 35% of all post-neonatal deaths. Around a quarter of such cases are "Accidental Strangulation and Suffocation in Bed" (ASSB), while around two thirds are "Sudden Infant Death Syndrome" (SIDS) cases, unexplained after autopsy and review.

Co-sleeping represents a recurrent cause of preventable infant deaths. It is not the only contributing factor, however, with many more including: very young (or old) maternal age, smoking, substance abuse, inadequate pre-natal care, poor social supports and low socio-economic and educational status. Since the causes of such deaths are legion, the responses are, of necessity, multifactorial.

Louisiana has a number of programs intended to address our unacceptable numbers of infant deaths. They include the Nurse Family Partnership (which sends visiting nurses to first time high-risk Medicaid eligible mothers), New Beginnings with Volunteers of America (pregnancy testing, Medicaid applications centers, pregnancy education), Partners for Health Babies (connecting moms and babies to resources), Caring Choices (mental health services for addiction), United Way (resource guide for CENLA), Louisiana Breast Feeding Coalition (encouraging breast feeding with Ban the Bag and Baby Friendly Hospitals), 39 Week Delivery Policies, and various prenatal care programs (encouraged through HealthyLouisiana, electronic health record use, meaningful performance use, improvement measures, and engagement with local obstetricians. We owe it to our most vulnerable citizens, our infants, to reduce morbidity and mortality whenever and however possible.

LGBT/Q: NEW VOCABULARY, NEW PARADIGMS

Many years ago during a class in adolescent sexuality at the medical school at the Catholic University of Louvain in Brussels, Belgium, a distinguished professor declared, "*La sexualité est comme un arbre avec un seul tronc et des multiples branches*" (Sexuality is like a tree with a single trunk and many branches.) Our very human tendency to classify and separate, however, may lead to oversimplifications. Everything is not black or white, right or wrong, or gay or straight. There are always many shades of gray, especially where sexuality is concerned.

The controversies surrounding the use of bathrooms by transgender individuals have highlighted a growing awareness of sexual diversity in the general population. For those unfamiliar with the nomenclature, it can be a confusing world, indeed.

First, LGBT/Q stands for Lesbian, Gay, Bisexual, Transgender and Questioning (or Queer). Lesbian refers to women who are sexually attracted to other women. Gay traditionally refers to men attracted to other men with whom they may have sex. Bisexual, of course, covers people who are attracted and may have sex with both the same and opposite sex. Some people classify themselves as "pansexual."

Transgender refers to sexual identity that does not correspond with the "sex assigned at birth" (also sometimes called "biological sex.") Transgender is sub-classified into "transmen," or women who identify as men and "transwomen" or men who identify as women. Transgender individuals may or may not receive hormonal treatments or surgical modifications to align themselves with their chosen sexual identity. That sexual identity is not the same as sexual preference, or those individuals to whom the individual is sexually attracted. A transman, (a women who identifies as a man) may be sexually attracted to either men or women or both.

Queer (or Questioning), once considered a derogatory term for lesbians and gays, has been embraced by people who reject the notion of "binary sexuality," (i.e. only two sexes.) Queer (or Questioning) becomes a blanket term for those have a certain sexual plasticity without being strictly bisexual. Their sexual orientation and identification may vary.

Controversy has swirled around the rights associated with all of these diverse sexual variations, notably with respect to the use of public bathrooms. In addition, regardless of the increased social acceptance of the LGBT/Q population over the last decades, sexual variations can still generate problems of social acceptance and self-esteem in some individuals. Increased levels of anxiety, depression, suicide, substance abuse and sexually transmitted diseases may accompany non-traditional sexual choices. Lesbian women, however, enjoy the lowest rates of sexually transmitted disease.

Beyond these "simple" classifications listed above, there also remains considerable sexual plasticity, especially among adolescents struggling to establish a sexual identity. Adolescents, filled with hormones, are biological adults while still "undeveloped frontal lobe children." The frontal lobes, responsible for reasoning and notions of delayed gratification, are not completely developed until twenty-five years of age. This de-synchronization between impulsive sexual behavior and delayed adult reasoning creates a propensity for experimentation and a minefield for high-risk behaviors with all of their undesirable outcomes.

How do we approach this new world of sexual diversity? First, we must educate ourselves about sexual diversity. Second, we must educate our youth about sexuality and its consequences. Only then can we hope to decrease the horrible burden of sexual abuse, teen suicide and sexually transmitted diseases (including HIV) that ravages our state. In Louisiana, we have among the highest rates of teen suicide (sometimes associated with a crisis of sexual identity) and we are number one in the nation in rates of syphilis and number two among states for chlamydia and gonorrhea and number three for HIV (primarily in individuals between 15 and 25 years of age). These grim statistics vary from year to year, but Louisiana has remained in the top five states for STDs and HIV for decades.

LBGT/Q or straight, all sexuality entails both benefits and risks and we must be informed about both. We must remember the distinction between sex at birth, sexual identity and sexual orientation when dealing with those in the LBGT/Q community. Ignorance is not bliss and silence is not golden.

LOCK 'EM UP

Every year there are a number of avoidable child and adolescent deaths due to two equally dangerous products: guns and controlled prescription medications. Both are legal and both can be lethal. Most of the deaths from guns are the result of children playing with loaded weapons or adolescent suicides. Both types of deaths are equally preventable when weapons are locked up.

No one will deny that America is awash with guns (88/100 people first in the world and far exceeding number 2, Yemen with 54.8/100 people). Americans, who represent less than 5% of the world's population, own over half of the world's firearms. Ownership of firearms in the U.S. has increase by 71% since 1994, with a 38% increase in the number of guns. Over 400,000 guns are stolen every year.

Guns kill over 1,300 U.S. Children every year. Gunshot wounds require the hospitalization of over 16 children in the U.S. daily. Older children (13 to 17) were more than 12 times more likely to die of firearm injuries than those below 12 years of age. In those in those 17 or less, 53% of the deaths were homicides, 38% suicides and 6% were accidental. Boys (82% of the victims) are more likely to die from gun-related violence than girls. Children's firearm deaths varied from state to state with Louisiana in the top, along with Colorado. Louisiana also toped the list for firearm related youth homicides, with African-Americans paying a disproportionate price. Louisiana was not among the top states in youth suicides.

Over 19 children a day are treated in emergency rooms for gunshot wounds and 16 of those are hospitalized. Among injuries, most were from assaults (71%), 21% were accidental and a small percentage (3% or less) was related to other causes. Besides the grief and sorrow related to unnecessary deaths, hospitalization related gunshot wounds cost over $700 million/year.

Recommendations for improvement of this unacceptable situation vary from simple to complex. Fierce opposition to gun control has paralyzed attempts to limit access to even the most lethal weapons, such as assault rifles. Attempts to enforce stricter controls become mired in emotional debates about the right to bear arms despite the horrific consequences of our firearm-saturated society.

Domestic violence and mental health issues, when associated with gun ownership (or access in the case of children and adolescents) can easily degenerate into murder or suicide. African-American youth die more often from gun-related homicides than motor vehicle accidents (the leading cause among White youth.) A lock box or gun safe should be mandatory in any home with a firearm, especially those with young children or adolescents. Smart guns that will only unlock for the designated user would also be useful. Last, but not least, banning assault rifles, with no possible civilian application, as well as devices to modify them in automatic weapons, would be useful in reducing deaths.

Easy access to firearms, promoted by powerful manufacturing interests, has disturbing parallels with the use of opioids in all age groups. Opioid use exploded over the last four decades, in parallel with narcotic-related deaths. Drug companies promoted the use of supposed "non-addictive" synthetic opioids and encouraged the use of pain as the "fifth vital sign." This helped fuel access to opioids in innumerable households where some of these products fell in the hands of children and adolescents.

Besides accidental overdoses, the inappropriate use of prescription opioids has fueled abuse in adults and young people. National campaigns to insure the proper storage of controlled substances have saturated the airways. Volatile adolescents, so prone to high-risk behavior of all types, can fall victim to substance abuse, gun violence or both. Pill parties use a combination of stolen medications to inebriate young people, sometimes with fatal results.

As for controlled medications, the parents have usually received a prescription from their doctor for a host of real and imaged ailments. Their use has increased dramatically over the last decades, driven by a combination of patient demand, compounded by marketing. The result has been an increased availability of these substances in homes across the United States. Adolescents, notorious for their lack of judgment, coupled with erratic and impulsive behavior, often experiment with prescription drugs found in their parent's medicine cabinet. Adolescent parties, known as "cocktail pill parties," involve the use of narcotic pain relievers, tranquillizers, and sleep agents, which are all put in a bowl and then ingested by the handful, often accompanied by alcohol. The results, much as with inappropriate gun use, can be fatal.

So parents, why take a chance? Lock up your guns and lock up your controlled substances (or destroy them), especially if they are no longer needed. Changes in physician practice standards should include limiting when opioids are used and the quantity and number of renewals, if any. Both guns and opioids can both be useful, even necessary, but not in the hands of children and adolescents. If adults must own guns and must use narcotic medications, make sure both are locked away securely. As adults, we can always choose to kill ourselves, but we should never be willing to participate, even unwittingly, in the massacre of innocent children.

MOTOR VEHICLE DEATHS IN INFANTS AND CHILDREN AND AGE-APPROPRIATE CHILD RESTRAINTS

The CDC examined motor vehicle deaths among children in the U.S. from 2006 to 2011. Every child's death is an extraordinary tragedy, but when they are preventable, the death becomes an unbearable burden to survivors and a horrific loss to society.

Motor vehicle deaths in children in the U.S. (1.9/100,000) are about double those in other high income European states (0.9/100,000). It has been established that rear-facing child safety seats to age 2, forward-facing child safety seats to age 5, booster seats to age 8 and adult seatbelts in the back seat to age 13 and beyond all reduce deaths in motor vehicle accidents by at least 35%. Despite laws requiring child safety seats in all states, age requirements vary and only 2% of children nationwide are required by law to have child safety seats and booster seats up to age 8.

While only 2% of children and infants are observed to be unrestrained in community studies, unrestrained children and infants represent 22% of deaths in motor vehicle accidents. The group of unrestrained infants and children varies with ethnic groups, with 90% of restraint use in Whites, 85% among Hispanics and 80% among African-Americans. Sadly, the death rates among African-American and Hispanic children are significantly higher than Whites. This relationship can be better correlated with poverty rather than race, since traumatic injuries among children with Medicaid exceed those among infants and children with private insurance. As with other health issues, outcomes can be correlated with insurance type.

Stricter and more uniform laws requiring rear-facing, correctly installed safety seats to age 2, forward facing children safety seats to age 5, and boosters in the back seat to age 8 would do a lot to decrease needless deaths. Since older children do what they see and what they are told, use of seat belts by adolescents and adults is crucial. Add to this a comprehensive education and safety seat distribution program and most tragic vehicle-related infant and child deaths could be avoided.

Vital Signs: Restraint use and motor vehicle occupant deaths rates among children aged 0-12 years. United States, 2002-2011. CDC. MMWR. Feb 7, 2014. 63(05); 113-118.

TEEN PREGNANCY IN THE UNITED STATES: WHERE WE STAND

Significant progress has been made in reducing teen pregnancy in the United States over the last two decades years. The number of births per 1,000 teens between 15 and 17 years of age dropped by 67% from 1991 (51.9/1,000) to 2012 (17/1,000). Proportionally, the greatest drop occurred in the 15 year olds (70%) as compared to the 16 (65%) and 17 year olds (61%). While good news, the rates of teenage pregnancy remain high in the U.S. (31.3/1,000 live births), when compared with other industrialized countries (24/1,000 in the U.K. and only 4/1,000 live births in the Netherlands). Teen births are particularly high in Louisiana at 45.1/1,000 births, although better than Arkansas and Mississippi at 50/1,000 live births. Among all U.S. teens that become pregnant, there are significant differences between races, with Hispanics (25.5/1,000 teens) and African-Americans (21.9/1,000) several times higher than whites (8.4/1,000) and Asians (4.1/1,000).

The declines in teen pregnancies in the U.S. are attributed to a combination of decreased sexual activity (23%) and changes in contraceptive methods (77%). The latter included increased use of highly effective contraceptives such as LARCs (Long-Acting Reversible Contraceptives), which include both intra-uterine devices (IUDs: *Paragard*®, *Mirena*®, *Skyla*®, *Liletta*® *and Kyleena*®) and implantable devices (*Nexplanon*®). Even though most sexually active teens (92%) used some form of contraception, they generally use condoms, which are often used incorrectly and are one of the least effective contraceptive methods.

Most young teens (15-17 years of age) that become pregnant are in high school, but only 38% of them will go on to complete their secondary education. Over 80% of teens that become pregnant had not received adequate sex education in school (despite the fact that 85% of parents supported its inclusion in the curriculum) and around 25% had never spoken to their parents about any form of contraception, including abstinence. That being said, among sexually active teens, over half (58%) had visited a healthcare provider for reproductive health services. Despite these visits, over 80% of teen pregnancies are still unintended, substantially higher than the surprising 50% rate among all U.S. women (which is higher than the estimated 40% rate or less among women in other developed countries.)

So what can be done about reducing teen pregnancy even further? Parents, guardians and caregivers can talk to teens about sexuality, including contraception, keep teens out of high risk situations (unsupervised parties with alcohol consumption), and being very aware of social media influences on adolescents. Increased use of LARCs (Long-Acting Reversible Contraception), including intrauterine devices and implantable rods (in the upper arm) would go a long way to decreasing unintended pregnancies, especially because teenagers may use other methods incorrectly or only intermittently.

Healthcare providers should encourage delayed sexual activity in adolescents, but also offer open, honest, convenient, confidential and respectful services to them. The substantial risks of STDs (including HIV), especially in Louisiana (which ranks in the top 4 U.S. states for STDs and HIV rates), should be stressed, with recommendations for safe sex practices among sexually active teens. Adolescents should discuss these matters openly with parents, healthcare professionals and educators (a particular challenge in Louisiana) and recognize their responsibilities in preventing unintended pregnancies and STDs, both of which can be life-altering experiences.

TEENAGE PREGNANCIES: OPPORTUNITIES FOR IMPROVEMENT

While teen births have declined in the U.S. over the last decade, over 273,000 infants are born each year to women 15 to 19 years of age. Teen births have immense economic, social and health consequences to the mother. Teen mothers often have lower education attainment, resulting in decreased salary expectations and lifelong earning potentials.

While abstinence is laudable, 43% of teenage girls have had sexual intercourse and even more have participated in oral sex. The latter is often not even considered true "sex" by many teens despite the fact that it exposes participants to STDs that are particularly omnipresent in Louisiana.

Teenagers are waiting longer to have intercourse and most (86%) use some form of contraception. Unfortunately, the methods available are very different in their effectiveness. Condoms, the most frequent choice of teens, are often used incorrectly and their use is associated with pregnancy in 18/100 women.

Birth control pills, another common choice, can be easily forgotten by busy teens and 9/100 women will become pregnant. Though twice as effective as condom use, birth control pills are still much less effective than LARCs (Long Acting Reversible Contraception). LARCs include both IUDs (Intra-Uterine Devices) and implants (Nexplanon®).

IUDs must be inserted directly into the uterus in a minor medical procedure performed by a doctor or a trained nurse practitioner. IUDs can be non-hormonal (copper), which last up to ten years. They can also be hormone containing and last from three to five years depending on the brand.

Women who choose a copper IUD will experience no changes in their normal periods. Hormonal IUDs, on the contrary, can cause infrequent spotting or suppress periods altogether. There can also be some temporary cramping following insertion. Otherwise IUDs pose few problems and are one of the most popular forms of birth control internationally.

The implant (Nexplanon ®) is a small progestin-filled tube that is inserted in the arm using a special device. Local anesthesia is required, which can be no more painful than a bee sting. The insertion itself is painless. The device causes no discomfort, nor any physical limitations. The implant lasts three years and can be removed sooner if problems develop or fertility is desired. This device is especially popular in university age women, especially if they have been previously receiving the progestin shot (DepoProvera ®) and are familiar with its pros and cons.

DepoProvera® or "the shot" must be given every 13 weeks in an intramuscular injection. Like the implant and hormonal IUDs, the shot results in irregular spotting or even cessation of menstrual bleeding altogether, a real plus for many women.

IUDs and the implant are both highly effective, with only 1/100 women becoming pregnant. They are 9 times more effective than the pill and 18 times more effective than condom use. While LARC use has increased over the years, only 7% of women choose these highly effective methods. Their use is particularly low in the South where LARC use is less than 5%.

Central Louisiana does distinguish itself by a higher LARC usage than other regions of the state. Promotion of these methods and same-day insertions at health units has resulted in CENLA having the highest absolute and highest per capita use of LARCs compared with the eight other public health regions.

As healthcare providers, we must recognize that teens, by their very nature, are impulsive risk takers. We must be sure that all teens are educated as to the hazards of teen pregnancy and STDs as well as the methods available to them should they choose to have sex. Precocious sexual activity and promiscuity should be discouraged since no form of birth control (even condoms) completely protects against STDs/HIV, so prevalent here in Louisiana.

A study by the Louisiana Public Health Institute confirmed that over 85% of Louisiana parents support the inclusion of comprehensive STD and contraceptive education in schools. Despite this fact, mandatory, meaningful sex education exists in very few school districts in the state.

The decision to have sex and to have children should be an intelligent, informed choice, not the result of misinformation and impulsive risk taking, so prevalent in teenagers.

MEASLES: A RECURRENT THREAT

In 2014, a measles outbreak, radiating throughout the U.S. from an imported case at Disney World in Anaheim, California, captivated national attention. In February 2015, there were over 140 recorded cases, with potential for rising considerably higher. Although the beginning of this outbreak originated from the "Magical Kingdom," past outbreaks began in less colorful locations, but still had the same remarkable spread (over 600 U.S. cases in 2013 alone.)

Measles is one of a number of childhood diseases that can be successfully prevented with vaccinations. The MMR (Mumps-Measles-Rubella) vaccine, usually given at one year and four years of age, offers life-long protection to the recipients. Those born prior to 1957 are considered immune because of the widespread nature of the disease prior to the introduction of a highly effective vaccine.

Since most children are vaccinated, what are the problems peculiar to measles? First, measles was declared eradicated in the United States in 2000, which means there were no circulating indigenous cases. Worldwide, however, the situation is far different, with many areas of incomplete vaccination and on-going cases. Under these circumstances, imported cases are always possible, even inevitable.

Second, measles is only one of several highly contagious viruses that are truly air-borne. Many other infections are droplet borne (such as influenza or tuberculosis), but those droplets can only extend out approximately three feet at which point gravity pulls them to the ground where they are unlikely to cause infection. Measles, on the contrary, floats in the air and can do so for hours. Anyone entering in a room or public space where a measles-infected individual passed, can inhale the virus and become infected. In fact, if 100 unvaccinated people walked through a room where a measles patient had been in the recent past, 90 of them would come down with measles! There are only a few other such airborne viral threats. Smallpox was one of these, which has fortunately been eliminated.

Third, there is a growing reservoir of children in the U.S. who have not been vaccinated. Misguided and ill-informed parents exaggerate the risks of vaccination and minimize the risks of failure to vaccinate against measles and other diseases. Often they have never seen cases in their lifetimes (nor have many current physicians). In reality, measles, far from a harmless childhood disease, can result in pneumonia, encephalitis (inflammation of the brain) and death. Around 25% of U.S. citizens infected with measles will require hospitalization and 1/500 could die.

Because of these three facts (the overseas reservoir of cases, the highly contagious nature of the virus and the growing group of unvaccinated children in the United States) measles remains a serious threat. Vaccines can have some side effects, mostly mild and transitory, but the decision not to vaccinate ignores scientific evidence and defies common sense. No vaccination causes autism. So protect your children and others by vaccination; you owe it to your loved ones and to your community.

WHY DO BABIES AND CHILDREN DIE IN CENTRAL LOUISIANA?

In an effort to prevent infant and child deaths in Central Louisiana, a group of stakeholders and experts meets on a regular basis to review the cases in this region. Two separate groups, both sponsored by the Bureau of Family Health, perform this sad duty: Fetal-Infant Mortality Review and the Child Death Review. These panels are made up of doctors, law enforcement, public health personnel, educators, hospital providers and others, all with some special expertise and a willingness to explore the whys and hows of infant and child deaths.

Since 2012, 101 cases have been reviewed and discussed in Central Louisiana, 54 of them in infants less than one-year-old and 47 of them between one year and 15 years of age. Which infants and children are dying and what conclusions can be drawn, if any, about ways to prevent these tragic deaths?

More Whites (64%) than Blacks (35%) are represented, with more males (62%) dying than females (39%). The majority (75%) of deaths were among Medicaid recipients, perhaps not surprising in an economically depressed region and state. Most of the incidents (66%) occurred at home under nominal supervision (78%) with parents as caregivers (83%).

The vast majority of such cases undergo an investigation (89% by the police or sheriff's department) and they are accompanied by a formal coroner's report (99%). Almost half of the deaths occurred with the infant or child sleeping (58%) although 17% took place with the child playing and 16% as an occupant of a motor vehicle.

The cause of death varies with the age, of course, but globally, 20% resulted from motor vehicle accidents, 7% occurred from electrocution,

10% from drowning and 37% from asphyxia (smothering), while 5% resulted from a weapon. Among infants, 15% were classified as SIDS (Sudden Infant Death Syndrome) or SUIDS (Sudden Unexplained Infant Death Syndrome), while nearly 40% were attributed to unsafe sleeping habits (usually co-sleeping with parents with inappropriate bedding). ATVs caused 5% of deaths and substance abuse by the parents or other caregivers was present in 11%.

After this depressing litany of statistics, our obligations as citizens, officials and parents is to tease out the preventable causes among these infant and child deaths. Clearly, co-sleeping and substance abuse fall squarely as preventable factors. Drowning should also be eliminated through childhood education, as should the inappropriate use of motor vehicles, including ATVs. Seat belts and other child restraints clearly save lives if and when properly used. Weapons-related deaths (5%) and poisonings (3%) can also be eliminated by effective storage practices by parents and guardians.

Despite all the bad news, Central Louisiana can boast the lowest three-year (2014-2015-2016) infant mortality rates in Louisiana, although not below national standards. Our child death rates, while not the highest in the state, are still unacceptably elevated.

Although the Fetal-Infant Mortality Review group in the OPH Regions was suspended in 2018, the Child Mortality Review and the Community Action and Advisory Team continue to meet. Anyone interested in participating in the Community Action and Advisory Team should feel free to contact Mrs. Lisa Norman for inclusion in that group. Specific initiatives, whether they are directed toward infants or children, must be pursued in order to end preventable deaths in this vulnerable age group.

TOOTH DECAY AND DENTAL SEALANTS IN SCHOOL-AGED CHILDREN

By the age of 19, one in five children has tooth decay. Poverty plays an important role, with twice as many low-income children having cavities than their better off counterparts. When untreated, cavities lead to pain, problems chewing, speech difficulties and even learning problems. Parents of low-income families report one or more episodes of toothache in the last six months in 16% of their children. Such dentally challenged children miss more school and have lower grades than children with better dental health. Most tooth decay occurs in the molars (the permanent back teeth) and represents a serious and costly problem.

Poverty, as a social determinant of health, is difficult to address, but cavities are responsive to better dental care regardless of economic level, notably with the use of sealants. Sealants are an easy-to-apply plastic coating that covers small holes and cracks in the enamel that lead to tooth decay. Once applied, sealants reduce cavities by 81% in the first two years and 50% within four years of application. The seal remains effective almost a decade. Sealants have no down side and the application process is simple, effective and without side effects.

Sadly, this simple and effective treatment is woefully underutilized, especially among the population groups that would most benefit from it. Among children 6 to 11, only 43% have received an application of sealant. This drops to 38.7% among low-income children. Use of sealant is highest among White, better-educated families with higher incomes.

The use of sealants has increased from 2004 to 2014 from 31.1 to 43.6%. The increase was greatest among families with low incomes (16.2% increase) compared to higher-income children (8.8% increase). There was a corresponding decrease in tooth decay, which decreased 4.9% in low income children. It remained about the same with higher-income children.

While sealants helped both low and high-income children, only 60% of low-income children receive the treatment. This leaves around 6.5 million children untreated. These untreated children are three times more likely to develop significant decay in their first molars.

Sealants are cost-effective and the positive economic consequences become apparent within two years. This results in Medicaid savings as well as benefits from reduced pain, lower absenteeism and improved learning. A licensed dental professional, although not necessarily a dentist, must apply the sealant. Failure to undergo regular dental checkups plays a negative role. Low literacy levels, especially among non-English speaking households, also negatively effects dental care, especially sealant use.

School programs, while effective, are far from universal. Where available, they mostly use less expensive dental hygienists or other paraprofessionals to place the sealants rather than dentists. Fluoridation of water also prevents tooth decay. That, too, requires a community commitment to such programs, which are sometimes opposed by vocal, if ill-informed, activists. Fluoridation and sealants have synergistic positive effects.

Children and parents need to understand the importance of dental hygiene, regular dental visits, and the use of sealants. Adequate dental providers, insurance coverage, and the use of school-based sealant programs with dental paraprofessionals all increase the use of sealants with their positive short and long-term benefits. Let's embrace cost-effective dental sealant programs so all our children, rich and poor, will benefit in the long term.

Griffin, SO et al., Dental Sealant Use and Untreated Tooth Decay Among U.S. School Aged Children. MMWR, Oct 18, 2016; (Vol 65): 1-5.

PHARMACOLOGY

EXORBITANT MEDICAL COSTS: WHO'S REALLY TO BLAME?

There has been much recent name-calling about exorbitant medical costs associated with a lot of unjustified finger pointing. Rather than grandstanding, a careful look at the current situation might shed some light.

The cost of medical care in the U.S. defies reason. We spend almost $9,000 per person per year on medical care, with less being spent on young people and almost double that amount for those 65 and older and three times that on those 85 and older. Medical expenditures exceed 18% of the U.S. Gross National Product (GDP), almost twice the percentage of other developed countries. The total amount spent reaches a staggering three trillion dollars annually, dwarfing the amount spent on the military (4.5% of GDP vs. 18%).

This enormous economic pie is generated by a combination of private and public dollars that approach 40% each, with a smattering from other sources. This is a far different picture from other developed countries where public expenditures contribute from 80 to 95% or more of total healthcare costs.

Where does this three trillion dollars per year go? A huge chunk goes to inpatient hospital care (around 40%) and another big chunk goes to doctors (around 35%) and the rest goes to a combination of pharmaceuticals, home health, durable medical equipment and a host of other lesser items, including around 7% for administrative costs.

What do we get for all this money? Despite these enormous and disproportionate expenditures, the U.S. life expectancy and other key indicators of health (including infant and maternal mortality) lag behind all other developed countries. In short, we spend much more than other countries per capita and get much worse health outcomes. Sadly, the truth is that every system is perfectly designed to produce the results that it produces, however bizarre.

Increases in cost have been not been uniform over the years, but have favored new expensive technologies (notably imaging such as MRIs and CT scans, robotic surgery, specialized radiation techniques and advanced cardiac catheterization, to name but a few) and pharmaceuticals (such as immuno-biologicals, new diabetic treatments or new oral anticoagulants, among others.)

The cognitive skills associated with bedside diagnosis and time-consuming counseling have increased in cost (and reimbursement), but at nowhere near the pace of that for new technologies or medications. Preventive care and socio-economic interventions, while much more cost-effective for improved health outcomes, are far less glamorous and often not reimbursed at all.

We thus have a huge $3 trillion dollar pie of medical expenditures from which many people in the medico-industrial complex derive impressive incomes and yet our health outcomes languish behind countries that pay half as much per capita and far less in absolute terms.

This situation did not occur overnight, but has been the result of unrelenting increases in medical expenditures since the 1980's. Since per capita health expenditures tend to rise with a country's per capita incomes, it is normal that there have been increases over the last decades. This has occurred in all developed countries. But the rate of cost increases in the U.S. has exceeded that of all other developed counties. This phenomenon has, however, made certain individuals and corporate entities fabulously wealthy without a proportional increase in national health.

The U.S. has turned into a monumental international outlier for our cost/benefit ratio, which has clearly reached the point of diminishing returns. What does that mean? The "law of diminishing returns" states that increases in expenditures result in increasing returns only to a certain point. Beyond that, even massive increases in money spent result in only minimal improvements, a point we have clearly reached some time ago.

So who is really to blame for our woefully expensive and inefficient system that has developed over time into a complex public-private partnership? Policy makers and legislators at all levels have endorsed and promulgated the laws governing the current system. They have also ignored the worsening signs of an impending crisis for decades. The public also may demand perfect outcomes with minimal waiting times, while often ignoring simple preventive measures that will protect their health and prolong their lives (such as weight loss, tobacco cessation and appropriate vaccinations).

To blame any one individual, whether they be a public official or a private citizen, is foolish and self-serving. We all got into this mess together and now we all need to get out together. Public outcry and business objections to ever rising costs have contributed to an increased awareness of the crisis. They have also resulted in a number of initiatives toward cost containment and quality improvement (managed care, accountable care organizations, MARCRA related changes in Medicare reimbursement and the Affordable Care Act, or whatever follows it, to name but a few).

Legitimate attempts to achieve international standards of universal health insurance have often been met with hostility and derision, yet it remains the gold standard of health care. The real problem is not the goal of universal health insurance, but the fact that it becomes a national fiscal liability to extend our already extravagantly expensive medical care to everyone. The real culprit is not universal health insurance, but a grossly inefficient and horrendously expensive health care system.

We must decrease the size of the $3 trillion pie of health expenditures. Howls of opposition to any decrease come from everyone who benefits economically from the current system, notably our extensive medico-industrial complex (from health care providers to pharmaceuticals to medical malpractice attorneys, to name but a few). But a sustainable system that works to the benefit of all should be our common goal. Let's stop finger pointing and start working toward reforming the system that serves us so poorly from a national and sometimes an individual perspective.

THE TRIUMPH AND TROUBLE WITH
THE IMMUNO-BIOLOGICALS

Immuno-biologicals represent a new class of medications, used for a wide variety of conditions. They modulate the body's immune response in different ways to either enhance or reduce inflammation (thus their other name, "biological response modifiers.") In a sense, they continue the tradition of older anti-inflammatory medication, the most famous of which is aspirin. Traditionally, anti-inflammatory medications were classified into non-steroidal anti-inflammatories (or NSAIDS, including aspirin, ibuprofen, naproxen and others) and steroids (cortisone-like agents.) The latter have broad anti-inflammatory and immunosuppressive qualities, but also cause glucose intolerance, weight gain, susceptibility to infection, bone loss and other unpleasant side effects.

With increased scientific understanding of the inflammatory process, there has been a proliferation of agents that target very specific steps in that complex cascade. These immuno-biologicals have been approved and promoted for use in an astonishing array of diseases including psoriasis, rheumatoid arthritis, Crohn's disease, ulcerative colitis, multiple sclerosis, many types of cancers (kidney, melanoma, leukemia, and lymphoma) as well as other evolving indications.

These diverse agents include interferons (that inhibit cell growth), interleukins (that stimulate the immune system), colony stimulating factors (that promote healthy cell growth) and monoclonal antibodies (proteins that target specific cells or intracellular components.) Their diversity of action all leads to biological response modulation. Since they often dull the inflammatory response in some way, they can also predispose toward infections, notably tuberculosis. Screening tests for TB must be performed before many of them can be administered.

Since these medications are "new and effective," they are aggressively promoted in advertising to the general public (and to providers). They represent a change in therapeutic choices for the practitioners, but also a marketing challenge to drug companies. While effective, all of these new immune-biologics cost many times more than previous therapies.

Drug companies, anxious to recover research and development cost, market these medications aggressively to the general public. This direct-to-consumer marketing strategy (unlawful in almost all countries except the U.S., Brazil and New Zealand), encourages patients to consult with their physicians to receive the newest (and presumably best) therapy. Whether it costs pennies a month, as with many older drugs, or thousands of dollars as with new immuno-biologicals, cost is generally glossed over (especially in public advertising.) "Ask your doctor," remains the mantra.

The old dilemma of cost vs. benefit ratios bubbles up to the surface once more. For the insured individual, third party payers are often left to decide who should benefit and at what price. Similar questions arise for chemotherapy (sometimes with immuno-biologicals) whose impact on survival might be measured in days or weeks rather than in years.

Since the scientific name for many immuno-biologicals ends in "-ab," "-ib" or "-cept," the general consumer can sometimes get a clue about this new class of medications. Many patients must still often pay hefty co-pays on pharmaceuticals, so sticker shock might be added to your previous illnesses. A candid conversation with an informed medical provider should take place. Unfortunately, many, if not most, doctors remain woefully unaware of the true cost of treatments (as well as tests, procedures and hospitalizations), and drug marketers often scrupulously avoid the subject.

No other services besides medical costs have remained so opaque to consumers and providers alike, yet financial considerations must remain at least a part of the decision-making process for individuals and institutions. As an attending physician at Johns-Hopkins once told the residents, "You will never solve the national debt at the patient's bedside." While true, being aware of the real cost of medical care, including immuno-biologicals, can only enhance patient care.

Look for the "-ab," "-ib," or "-cept" ending on the scientific name of a drug and ask a few probing questions. How is it given (oral or injection)? Is it really better than older, cheaper medications? If so, what will it cost and can I afford it? Using the free app, GoodRx, can help you find the real cost of your prospective treatment and the cheapest source among the pharmacies. While you may not pay much out of pocket for an immuno-biological, there is no such thing as a free lunch and someone pays the pharmaceutical piper.

DIRECT ORAL ANTICOAGULANTS (DOACS)

Anticoagulants, substances that thin blood, have long been used in a number of medical conditions, notably atrial fibrillation and the prevention of deep venous thromboses. The gold standard for anticoagulation has long been warfarin (Coumadin®), a vitamin K inhibitor that blocks the production of certain key components of the very complex coagulation (clotting) cascade. Warfarin works well at inhibiting blood coagulation, "thinning blood," but it must be monitored to insure that the patient's blood is "not too thin and not too thick. This is accomplished by periodic blood tests (notably the INR and/or the Prothrombin Time or PT).

This so-called "therapeutic range" for warfarin anticoagulation is fairly narrow and the blood-monitoring interval might be as frequent as weekly or as long as a month or more. Many medications and foods can interfere with warfarin's actions and make the patient more susceptible to either bleeding or clotting. Sometimes catastrophic gastrointestinal or intra-cerebral bleeding can occur that can be life-threatening.

Warfarin does have the advantage of being reversible with the use of vitamin K (whose actions on clotting are inhibited by warfarin). This takes time, however, since the body must regenerate the warfarin-inhibited clotting components. Rapid reversal can be achieved with the use of I.V. fresh frozen plasma, which contains all of the clotting elements and is used in bleeding emergencies.

In order to make anticoagulation easier and safer, pharmaceutical companies have developed a number of new oral agents called Direct Oral Anticoagulants (DOACs) or sometimes called New Oral Anticoagulants (NOACs). These include dabigatran (Pradaxa®), Rivaroxaban (Xarelto®), apixaban (Eliquis®) and Edoxaban (Savaysa®). These new oral agents act at different points of the clotting cascade, making them equally effective as warfarin and somewhat easier to use. They do not require the regular blood tests associated with warfarin, and may be less prone to catastrophic bleeding events (either gastrointestinal or cerebral) depending on the particular drug.

Why then are these newer agents not universally proscribed as safe and effective alternatives to warfarin? There are two reasons. The first is that, until very recently, there was no medication that reversed the DOACs in cases of bleeding. One agent, dabigatran (Pradaxa®), now does have such a reversing agent (Idarucizumab or Praxbind®) and others are in development.

The second reason has been cost. While warfarin costs a mere $4 per month (not including the costs of lab tests), the DOACs all cost around $400 per month. This hundred-fold increase causes concern among payers, specifically insurers such as Medicare and Medicaid. Pharmaceutical companies have countered hesitancy about their use with extensive, aggressive direct consumer marketing, especially in those patients with atrial fibrillation. Direct patient marketing has proven effective in promoting the use of DOACs when the providers (a naturally conservative group) prove recalcitrant to prescribe them. Pharmaceutical companies are locked in a race against time to maximize the sale of their new, expensive drugs before competitors rush in to challenge them when their patents expire and cheaper generics are developed and introduced.

While NOACs are safe and effective, their use still raises the age-old medical problem of cost/benefit ratios. The tug of war between the patient, providers, payers and pharmaceutical companies plays out every day in doctors' offices, corporate boardrooms and even the halls of congress. Since the majority of those with atrial fibrillation are seniors, Medicare, with its ever rising costs, is a policy focal point for legislators.

Bringing up these new anticoagulant agents with your doctor can certainly be a useful starting point, but it might not be the end of the discussion. Meanwhile keep an eye on the NOACs, which might be a better choice for you, if you can afford them.

MRSA (METHICILLIN RESISTANT STAPH AUREUS) AND HEROIN: THE DOCTOR'S DILEMMA

Perhaps you are wondering what MRSA and heroin have in common and why either would pose a dilemma to a physician. What is this dilemma and what do these two seemingly very different things have in common?

MRSA (Methicillin Resistant Staphylococcus Aureus) is a germ that plagues health care providers and institutions. Staphylococcus aureus lives on skin and is found to varying degrees on most people. In itself, it is fairly harmless, but it can cause superficial wound infections in some individuals and life-threatening septicemia in others. Staphylococcus aureus was originally sensitive to penicillin, the miracle antibiotic of the mid-20th Century. Within a few years, however, some Staphylococcus strains had developed resistance to penicillin following its widespread use. What eventually resulted was a race over time between pharmaceutical companies and the germ. Staphylococcus developed resistance to a host of newly developed antibiotics, first methicillin, and subsequently a number of others. Now, especially virulent MRSA organisms (often found in health care facilities) are resistance to all but a few expensive antibiotics whose use is restricted to infectious disease specialists.

During this same time, MRSA moved from the hospital and nursing home out into the general community where it can be contracted by athletes and others. Both the hospital acquired and community acquired versions of MRSA can be combatted by measures of hygiene and what is called "antibiotic stewardship," or the judicious use of antibiotics, notably abstaining from their use unless it is really necessary.

Heroin seems like another topic entirely, and yet the heroin epidemic in the United States has largely grown out of the overuse of pain medications, prescribed by doctors for various conditions. Almost every heroin addict, of which there are hundreds of thousands, started with pain medications prescribed to him or her legally. When unfortunate individuals become addicted, alleviation of symptoms is achieved either through using more legally or illegally obtained prescription medications or switching to "street drugs," most commonly heroin because of its low cost and availability.

What MRSA and heroin have in common that they have their origins in the injudicious use of antibiotics in the one case and pain medications in the other. Since both are prescription medications, it requires a doctor to write the prescription in the first place. If doctors know the dangers posed by overuse of either antibiotics or pain medications, then why are they being over-prescribed? Therein lies the "doctor's dilemma."

A patient with an infection (often a cold or upper respiratory infection) often expects or demands an antibiotic as treatment. Sometimes it is justified, but often it is inappropriate. Viral infections do not respond to antibiotics and often run their course regardless of the treatment. The doctor must decide to spend twenty minutes going into a difficult discussion of the importance of not giving unnecessary antibiotics (i.e. "antibiotic stewardship") or spend two minutes writing an antibiotic prescription that may hypothetically contribute to developing a resistant germ. From a purely economic standpoint, twenty minutes vs. two minutes is a no-brainer. In addition, a disgruntled patient often goes to another provider to get the antibiotics they think they need. And heaven forbid that the patient worsens without antibiotics and then develops a bacterial infection as a complication. The doctor becomes subject to litigation for "failing to diagnosis and treat."

Pain medications pose the same dilemma. A patient with a low pain tolerance, especially who has been previously treated with highly effective (and highly addictive) pain medications, will often request a specific brand of narcotic pain medication. It takes the doctor twenty minutes (or more) to explain the dangers of narcotic use and two minutes to write a prescription. The doctor also knows that the patient can and will seek another more compliant provider if they are refused. Fortunately, doctors can query Louisiana's Prescription Monitoring Program (PMP) to track narcotic medication use, although it is not required for regular physicians to do so at every visit at this time.

So the doctor confronts and resolves the dilemma as best he or she can. Do they want to spend the additional time to withhold antibiotics and pain medications, or do they capitulate and do the wrong thing from an ethical and medical standpoint? The proliferation of resistant organisms and the epidemic of heroin use across the United States speak for themselves. Aggravating the doctor's situation is the ubiquitous expansion of "Patient Satisfaction Surveys." Pleasing patents is often the condition for continued employment and advancement for employed physicians (of which there are more and more). While there is nothing wrong with being a pleasant, helpful, informative doctor, there are times when not giving the requested treatment or test is the ethical and medically correct thing to do. Patient satisfaction, however, may plummet.

Patients and physician are both complicit in the abuse of antibiotics and the abuse of addictive pain killing medications. Since we should be partners (and not adversaries) in health care, it remains to both the medical community and the larger patient community to understand that sometimes withholding antibiotics and narcotic pain medication is the right thing to do. Let's all be part of the solution and not part of the problem.

OSTEOPOROSIS: AN UPDATE

Osteoporosis literally means "porous bones." In medical terms, osteoporosis refers to bones with "compromised strength that predisposes to increased risk for fracture." Bone strength is a product of bone density and bone quality, both of which need to be in good shape. No one should underestimate the importance of osteoporosis. Around 53.6 million older U.S. adults have frank osteoporosis or low bone mass at the femoral neck (the hip) or lumbar spine (lower back). This represents an enormous problem because 1 out of 2 postmenopausal women and 1 out of 5 older men will have an osteoporotic-related fracture in their lifetime. Hip fractures, already an enormous medical issue in the elderly, are expected to double or triple by 2040 due to the aging U.S. population. Currently, there are over 300,000 people over 65 hospitalized for a hip fracture each year with an average orthopedic cost of $26,000/case, not counting subsequent rehabilitation. The estimate for total hip fracture related costs exceeds $12 billion/year.

To know if you have osteoporosis, you need to undergo a bone densitometry determination. Who should be tested and how often are the critical questions. The United States Preventive Services Task Force (or USPSTF) recommends screening all women 65 years or older. Postmenopausal women (aged 50-64) should be screened if they have had a fracture as an adult, have rheumatoid arthritis or other disease causing bone loss, take certain bone-weakening medications (such as steroids), or who have a 10-year fracture risk greater than a 65 year old women (as determined by a Z-score, explained below).

As for men, the USPSTF says there is "insufficient evidence" (an "I") to recommend systematic screening in men although the National Osteoporosis Foundation recommends screening men over 70 years of age.

Men with a 10-year risk for an osteoporotic fracture greater than that of a 65 year old woman without risk factors should also be screened.

What exactly are risks for fracture? They include an extensive list of items: low bone mineral density, advanced age, prior fracture, smoking and low body weight. Other risk factors, related to increased falls include poor vision, dementia, weakness, poor mobility, sedatives and narcotics, excessive alcohol (>2 drinks/day) and extreme frailty. There are also a host of medical conditions predisposing to osteoporotic fractures such as hyperthyroidism, hyperparathyroidism, diabetes mellitus, chronic liver disease, renal failure, rheumatoid arthritis, malabsorption and gastric bypass surgery, among others. Lastly, there are many medications that contribute to potential osteoporosis, notably steroids, anticonvulsants, glitazones and SGLT-2 inhibitors (for diabetes), proton pump inhibitors (antacids), some cancer medication and some serotonin receptor inhibitors (used for depression).

The only screening test that satisfies World Health Organization diagnostic criteria is the dual-energy x-ray absorptiometry (or DEXA) determined at the hip or lumber spine. The result is usually a "T-Score" or bone density compared to that of a normal young adult of your sex. A T-score of -1 and above is normal, from -1 to -2.5 shows osteopenia (pre-osteoporosis) and -2.5 and below indicates osteoporosis. (Z-Scores are used in some circumstances and compare people of the same age, sex, weight and ethnic origin. Below -2 indicates abnormal bone loss and should be treated.) There is also a "Vertebral Fracture Assessment" (VFA) that looks for vertebral fractions picked up incidentally or at the same time as a DEXA exam.

Frequency of appropriate screening has been evolving over time. Currently, the recommendation for screening in untreated older women (postmenopausal over 65 years old) is every 15 years for women with base-line T-Scores between -1 and -1.49, every 5 years for T-Scores between -1.5 and -1.99, and yearly for those with T-scores between -2 and -2.49.

Treatment can include bisphosphonates, denosumab or teriparatide, and should be offered to all frankly osteoporotic adults and to postmenopausal women or men under 50 if they have a T-Scores between -1 and -2.5 and a 10-year probability of hip fracture over 3% or a probability of any ostoeoporotic fracture over 20%. Without going to in excessive detail about osteoporosis treatments, the options include biphosponates (alendronate, risendronate, ibandronate and zoledronic acid), terparatide and denosumab. Biphosphonates inhibit the actions of osteoclasts (bone cells that dissolve bone) and come in daily or weekly oral forms or IV forms that can be given every 3 months or even every 12 months. Terparatide (given subcutaneously as a daily injection) alters bone metabolism as well as intestinal and renal calcium and phosphate absorption. Denosumab, which also inhibits osteoclast formation (bone absorbing cells), is given subcutaneously every 6 months.

Each of these three categories of treatments has its own extensive lists of warnings and side effects, including osteonecrosis of the jaw for bisphosphonates and denosumab, although the incidence (new cases) is extremely low (1/10,000 to 1/100,000). Treatment duration remains controversial, but after 3 to 5 years, a check for interval fractures, a new DEXA scan and vertebral height during the treatment period are warranted. A "drug holiday" after 3-5 years may be appropriate, and appears that a five-year limit may be recommended as well. As always, informed discussions with your internist or rheumatologist are mandatory due to the dire consequences of osteoporosis and the complexities of its treatment.

DIRECT TO CONSUMER ADVERTISING OF PHARMACEUTICALS

Direct-to-Consumer Advertising (DTCA) for pharmaceuticals is omnipresent on television in the United States. It is, in fact, permitted in only three places in the world besides the U.S.: New Zealand, Brazil and the City of Hong Kong. Although it seems to have been around forever, Direct-to-Consumer Advertising was restrained prior to 1997 at which time the Food and Drug Administration relaxed its regulations. Since then, spending on direct advertising has spiked from $1.1 billion in 1997 to $4.2 billion in 2005. It now represents over 12% of the $60 billion or more spent on pharmaceutical marketing every year, or over $7.2 billion.

Perhaps it is not a coincidence that the U.S. drug promotional spending per capita is the highest in the world. Although Americans do not consume more medications per capita, the selection of medications is skewed to those newer, more expensive medications that are the target of intense marketing. Americans spend around $1,000 per person per year on medications, around 30% more than those in other developed countries. Costs for some popular medications may be double or triple that of the same medications in Western Europe.

The vast amount of money spent on Direct-to-Consumer Advertising reflects not only shifts in regulatory supervision (or lack thereof), but also fundamental changes in health care delivery that occurred over the last decades. The advent of managed care brought with it fixed formularies. Doctors were given lists of medications that patients under a particular managed care plan could be prescribed without incurring "non-formulary" co-payments. That meant that doctors could simply default to the drug formulary for choices, leaving the managed care organizations to negotiate with the pharmaceutical companies for better deals.

Direct-to-Consumer Advertising meant that the consumer (no longer just the prescriber) became the target of intense pressure, in this case to "talk to your doctor" about a particular medication, often the newest and more expensive product. While there is some educational component to the advertising, the high cost of the advertised products (as compared with generics or pre-existing treatments) is not discussed.

So does Direct-to-Consumer Advertising work? Yes, at least for the pharmaceutical industry! There was a 34.2% increase in prescription rates of DTCA promoted drugs between 1998 and 1999 alone (compared to a 5.1% increase among non-DTCA promoted drugs during the same period.) For every $28 spend on DTCA, at least one patient will be prompted to see their doctor to ask about an advertised medication. A Kaiser Foundation report stated that 44% of patients received the DTCA medication they requested after a medical visit. Around 47% of doctors felt significantly pressured to prescribe the new medication even if there were questions about safety, efficacy or cost.

The very powerful Pharmaceutical Research and Manufacturers of America (PhRMA) defends the practice of Direct-to-Consumer Advertising as a way to inform and engage the public in medical care. They also claim that DTCA enhances research and development, competition and results in decreased pharmaceutical costs. Little evidence supports such claims. Pharmaceutical companies increased research and development costs by 59% from 1997 to 2001 alone, but they increased drug advertising by 145% during the same period.

In the end, it remains the consumer's responsibility to sift through the hype and help make an informed decision. The Latin admonition "Caveat Emptor" (Buyer Beware) still holds true today. The constant barrage of advertisements, whether they are for medications, automobiles or attorneys, should only be one small factor in decision making. Remember, however, that if you bring up that new, expensive medication you saw on television at your next appointment, your doctor is likely to prescribe it. The new medication may increase your health, but it will certainly increase cost to your insurance provider.

When you see a medication that is advertised on television, go on the free app, GoodRx, and find out the cost at your local pharmacies. Warning: It may give you palpitations.

PREVENTIVE CARE

CHANGING GUIDELINES FOR HYPERTENSION AND HYPERCHOLESTEROLEMIA

For those who are interested in preventive care, which should be everyone, there has been some comfort and consistency in recognizing and achieving goals suggested by your physician. These are not arbitrary goals, but the result of recommendations produced by expert panels from distinguished organizations (notably the American College of Cardiology, the American Heart Association and the National Heart, Lung, and Blood Institute.) Since 2003, the JNC (Joint National Committee, comprised of representatives of the above-mentioned groups) has made recommendations for blood pressure control. Everyone, both patients and physicians, formerly recognized that the upper acceptable limit for the systolic (top blood pressure) was 140 and the diastolic (lower blood pressure) was 90.

The latest JNC 8 recommendations raised the upper acceptable systolic pressure to 150 in non-diabetic, non-chronic kidney disease who are 60 years old or older. There were also more specific recommendations about the initial choice of medications in Whites (thiazide diuretics, calcium channel blockers, ace-inhibitors or angio-tension blockers) vs. Blacks (thiazide diuretics and calcium channel blockers). If blood pressure is NOT achieved in one month, increased doses or additional medication are suggested. If over three medications together are not successful in achieving blood pressure control, referral to a hypertension specialist is recommended.

Although all of this may seem rather academic, apparently 29% of the guideline writers dissented in promulgating these current JNC-8 recommendations. Blood pressure, just as its treatment, has proven a moving target as the upcoming JNC-9 recommendations attest. There are good indications that the threshold for blood pressure will, in fact, by lowered to 130/80 for all adults as recommended by the American Heart Association. Other major medical groups may follow suit. As they say, "stay tuned."

Similar issues have rocked the world of cholesterol guidelines. For some time, the goal of a LDL (low density lipoprotein or "bad cholesterol level") of 100 mg/dl or less was the standard recommendation (Adult Treatment Panel III). After decades of statin use and a series of major medical studies, experts from some of the same organizations (American College of Cardiology and the American Heart Association) have abandoned use of this figure. They have established four groups of primary and secondary prevention patients targeted for treatment with either high-intensity or moderate-intensity statins.

Group (1) includes patients with established atherosclerotic heart disease. Group (2) is those with LDL-cholesterol levels of greater than or equal to 190 mg/dl. Group (3) includes diabetics between 40 and 75 years of age with LDL levels between 70 and 189 mg/dl with NO evidence of vascular disease and Group (4), those without diabetes or vascular disease with LDL levels between 70 and 189 mg/dl WITH a 10-year risk of atherosclerotic cardiovascular disease equal or exceeding 7.5%.

Specific LDL-cholesterol goals are not recommended, rather percentage decreases of 50% in Groups 1 & 2 (using high-intensity statins) and 30% to 49% in Groups 3 & 4 (using moderate-intensity or high-intensity statins, depending on the level of risk.) To determine 10-year risk, there is a global risk assessment tool developed by the panel and available at the American Heart Association website.

Why the changes? The panel, using the aggregate of available scientific studies, hoped to achieve better outcomes in specific groups. Achieving a fixed goal of 100 mg/dl LDL across the board was apparently over-treating some and undertreating others. These changes are really an attempt to equilibrate risk and benefits, based on available research.

Making changes among physicians and patients alike is akin to changing the course of the Titanic. There will be much resistance from both groups, especially when the new recommendations appear so much more complex than the older ones. Do not be surprised, however, if your doctor mentions these changes and adjusts either your blood pressure treatment or statin doses accordingly. This may include removing several ineffective drugs, including fibrates, niacin and ezetimibe (Zetia®), thus simplifying your medication regimen, or perhaps re-adjusting or eliminating one of your blood pressure medications. If your physician does not mention the changes, feel free to ask about them.

DOMESTIC VIOLENCE IN LOUISIANA

For reasons probably related to poverty and low educational attainment, Louisiana has been plagued by a persistent problem of domestic violence. In this respect, it is no different than the United States as a whole where 1 women in 3 in the U.S. reports being a victim of domestic violence at least once in her lifetime. This comes to over 5,000,000 individuals a year (larger than the entire population of Louisiana). Rape is one manifestation of domestic violence and 20% of women and 1/70 men have reported being raped in their lifetime. Women between the ages of 16 to 24 are four times more likely to be raped than other age groups. Of these rapes, more than half were acquaintances (especially dates, when 57% of rapes occur). Around 27% of the victims did not realize they were raped and 42% do not report the episode.

Sadly, domestic violence, which represents 21% of all reported crimes in Louisiana, can escalate to murder and our state was the 2nd highest in the U.S. in its partner murder rates in 2014 (30.3/100,000 inhabitants). One domestic violence murder has occurred in every parish in Louisiana from 1997 to 2009 and they continue to occur. In CENLA, the Rapides Foundations reported that 13.8% of adults had been "hit, slapped, pushed, kicked, or hurt in some way by an intimate partner." This happened least in Catahoula, Allen and Winn Parishes (6.5 to 8.1%), and most in LaSalle, Natchitoches, Rapides and Vernon Parishes (14.9 to 16.3%). Among victims, low income, Black women suffered the highest levels.

The cycle of violence is especially severe, as mentioned, among women and girls who are vulnerable due to endemic dependence and long-standing cultural stereotypes of male dominance. Violence tends to spill over to other family members and can include child abuse or elderly abuse as well.

Beyond the obvious medical costs of domestic violence, the social costs are enormous including lost wages, lost educational attainment, unwanted pregnancies, low self-esteem, depression and suicide. Women often blame themselves rather than their perpetrators and can feel humiliated and powerless to prevent violence or extricate themselves from the situation.

Rapes or other violence often goes unreported, as mentioned earlier, or worse yet, the victims presented to the hospital ER only to be charged for the medical costs of the exam and sexual assault work up. Fortunately, that sad state of affairs came to an end with legislation that prevented hospitals from charging victims of sexual assault for their work-up. In addition, there are various local groups including the Faith House, United Way, CASA and others who are collaborating to reduce our inappropriately high levels of domestic violence and abuse in CENLA. There is currently a resource center on the grounds of the former Huey P. Long Hospital to serve the needs of abused women (and men), the Family Justice Center. It serves as a one-stop shop for physical, emotional and legal needs of victims of domestic abuse.

Although often hidden behind closed doors, the disgrace of domestic violence, both physical and psychological, should be exposed to the light of day. If you are a victim of abuse, including rape or date rapes, or a witness to domestic violence, please report them! We all have a responsibility to stop this plague in our society. Reporting child abuse is already a legal obligation for health care providers, clergy, emergency personnel, teachers, social workers and others. By eliminating individual occurrences, we just might be able to improve our regional and state statistics. Reducing or eliminating domestic violence may be just the top of a larger, more sinister iceberg of social and economic issues, but since they are all related, at least we can make a start.

Report domestic violence at 1-888-4121-1333 (Louisiana Coalition Against Domestic Violence and FAITH HOUSE.)

Report Child Abuse and Neglect to Dept. of Child and Family Services (DCSF) at 1-855-4LA-KIDS or 1-855-452-5437.

HEALTH SCREENINGS:
BENEFITS AND DANGERS

Ignorance is bliss? Or is it, and if so, when? Some people adopt an attitude that what they don't know can't hurt them. Alas, the ostrich attitude is not helpful, especially when HIV testing, blood pressure, cholesterol levels and breast or colon cancers are concerned. Yet the situation is far from being simple. Some screenings, especially in the right target group, bring positive benefits to the patients. Other screenings, however, can engage the patient in a host of expensive, dangerous and useless medical procedures that cause more harm than good.

Most people are aware of commercial screening companies that come to a local church or a medical provider-sponsored health fair. But are the proposed tests really indicated and what are their benefits? Fortunately, there is the United States Preventative Services Task Force (USPSTF), an independent organization of highly qualified professionals, who examine the science behind the testing to help answer those questions.

Commercial screening companies often propose the following tests: (1) Ultrasound screening of the carotid arteries, (2) EKG for "coronary heart disease" or "atrial fibrillation," (3) Ultrasound for abdominal aortic aneurysm, (4) Ankle-brachial index for peripheral arterial disease and (5) Heel bone densitometry for osteoporosis. Let's look at the evidence from the USPSTF.

"Stroke/Carotid Artery Screening" sounds like a good idea, but the USPSTF gives it a "D" grade ("Don't do it!") in asymptomatic adults. Why? The test should be reserved for those who have had symptoms or signs suggestive of arterial blockage (i.e. mini-strokes, dizziness, transient ischemic attacks, a "bruit" identified on physical exam, etc.) Screening patients without symptoms can result in many false positives (no real disease) and referrals for subsequent procedures, like angiography or even surgery, which may offer no benefit and entail significant cost and documented risks.

EKG's (electrocardiograms) are simple and effective in the right group, those with an irregular heartbeat (or cardiac symptoms). By taking your pulse, rhythm irregularities can be identified by your primary care doctor (or nurse or physician's assistant). In the general population, "abnormal EKG's" can be common and may or may not have any clinical significance. Subsequent testing (treadmills, heart ultrasounds, calcium scoring, or even heart catheterization) can all produce false positive results and each has its own expense and potential for problems. The USPSTF gives screening EKG's a "D" grade for diagnosing coronary heart disease in the general population.

While abdominal aortic aneurysms can be life threatening, they can be small and medically insignificant. The USPSTF only recommends "Abdominal Aortic Aneurysm Screening" tests in male smokers between 65 and 75 years of age ("B" Grade). It gets a "C" (neither recommended not discouraged) for non-smoking males between 65-75 years old and is NOT recommended ("D") for asymptomatic women.

This leads us to "Peripheral Arterial Disease Screening" with an ankle-brachial index. The test is simple, with a comparison of systolic blood pressures between the arm and ankle. A low index may indicate peripheral artery disease, presumably from blockage somewhere in the lower extremity. About 6% of adults over 40 can have a low index (<0.9), with higher percentages among diabetes and those with cardiovascular disease. The USPSTF gives this an "I" (insufficient evidence for recommendation.) Anyone with claudication (leg pain with walking) should certainly be tested, especially if they are diabetic or have known heart disease.

Finally, there is "Osteoporosis Risk Assessment." Osteoporosis is thinning of the bones and it can affect some post-menopausal women, increasing their risk for broken bones, notably hip and vertebral fractures. The USPSTF gives this screening a "B" for women over 65 and younger women with known risk factors (i.e. smoker, early menopause, hysterectomy, etc.). It receives an "I" (insufficient evidence for recommendation) for men.

David J. Holcombe

This is not an exhaustive review, but just an evaluation of some frequently performed commercial screening tests. It is best to look up any screening test on the USPSTF website where science, not monetary self-interest, dictates the decision making. In short, screenings can be good, but not necessarily every test for every individual every time.

http://www.uspreventiveservicestaskforce.org/recommendations.htm

PAP SMEARS AND PELVIC EXAM SCREENINGS: NEW GUIDELINES

Although women have long ago resigned themselves to the reality of a yearly pelvic exam, recommendations have changed in the last few years that should offer some relief. The U.S. Preventive Services Task Force (USPSTF) regularly reviews preventive health practices and aligns them with current research findings. Decisions include factors such as the sensitivity and specificity of screening exams as well as positive and negative predictive values, all somewhat complex statistical notions. There are ways, nonetheless, to evaluate the utility of any preventive test or procedure.

So where do we stand with the dreaded annual Pap smear. This test diagnoses cervical cancer, hopefully in its earliest stages. It has proven its effectiveness over the decades and has greatly reduced the rates of late stage cervical cancer in women. But when should it be started and how often should it be performed?

The USPSTF now recommends that Pap smears (cytology) be started in women at age 21. If the test is negative, the test can be repeated every 3 years (and not annually) until the woman reaches 30 years of age. From 30 to 65, the USPSTF recommends a combination test that includes the Pap smear (cytology) and a test for the human papillomavirus (HPV).

Why HPV testing? In fact, infection with HPV is necessary for the development of cervical cancer. It is a rare example of a cancer that depends on prior infection with a known virus to develop. You can certainly get HPV and not develop cervical cancer, but you cannot get cervical cancer without prior infection with HPV. Before 30 years of age, many women will be infected with HPV (something that can be prevented with appropriate vaccination), but most of them will clear the infection spontaneously without any particular treatment. After 30, this becomes much less common, so combining the Pap smear and the HPV test increases the accuracy of the testing.

The FDA recently approved the use of an HPV test as a primary test for cervical cancer. If the test is positive for HPV 16 or 18 (two cancer causing strains, identified in over 70% of cases of cervical cancer), then a follow-up colposcopy (a direct exam of the cervix) is recommended. When other high risk strains (around 14 of them) are identified, then a Pap smear follow up would be required to rule out cancer.

Although this sounds like more simplified testing method, the USPSTF still recommends against use of the HPV test alone or in combination in women 30 years of age and younger. And while speaking of age, between 30 and 65, a negative combination Pap-HPV test means that testing can be reduced to every 5 years (and not annually) after a negative test. After age 65, no further Pap smears are indicated if there is evidence of a normal exam with prior screening. In the absence of a high-grade precancerous or previous cervical cancer, women with a hysterectomy (with removal of the cervix) do not need to be screened.

In short, the recommendations for cervical cancer screening have become simplified and the tests reduced in number. In addition, the American College of Physicians has even recommended eliminating routine pelvic exams in asymptomatic, non-pregnant women of average risk during their annual wellness visits. They feel that the "harm outweighs any demonstrated benefits associated with the screening pelvic examination."

Women should arm themselves with the facts before going for their annual wellness exam or periodic cervical cancer screening. You might be in for a pleasant surprise and a less stressful and invasive visit.

http://www.uspreventiveservicestaskforce.org/

Qaseem, A et al. Screening Pelvic Examination in Adult Women : A Clinical Practice Guideline From the American College of Physicians. Ann Internal Medicine. 2014;161 (1):67-72.

PNEUMOCOCCAL PNEUMONIA AND THE NEW PNEUMOCOCCAL VACCINES

Streptococcus pneumonia is a common germ that causes a lot of avoidable problems. Although best known in adults as a cause of pneumonia, *Streptococcus pneumonia* can cause ear and sinus infections, meningitis and sepsis (blood infection) in both children and adults. It is estimated that Streptococcus results in over 4,000 of the 52,000 deaths attributable to pneumonia in adults each year.

Introduction of an effective vaccine against *Streptococcus* around 2000 has resulted in huge decreases in the rates of invasive pneumococcal disease (sepsis). Cases of documented sepsis from 1998 to 2006 in children less than 5 years old dropped from 100/100,000 to less than 20/100,000 (a five-fold decrease) and from 30/100,000 to less than 10/100,000 in adults 65-79 (a three-fold decrease). An even more dramatic drop in the same time period occurred in adults over 80 years old, with pneumonias dropping from 60/100,000 to less than 10/100,000 (a 6 fold decrease). In adults, the *Prevnar-13* reduced pneumococcal sepsis by 75% and non-septic pneumonia by 45% in a study of over 85,000 seniors. Pneumococcal vaccines work and they work very well in both adults and children.

There are two types of pneumococcal vaccines, the pneumococcal conjugate vaccine (PCV-13 or *Prevnar-13*®) and the pneumococcal polysaccharide vaccine (PPSV-23 or *Pneumovax-23*®). The number refers to the types of Streptococcal bacterial antigens in the vaccine. The latter, or *Pneumovax-23*® is limited to adults over 50 and certain high-risk younger patients with decreased immunity.

Children usually get *Prevnar-13*® doses at 2, 4 and 6 months of age, with the first dose as early as 6 weeks, and with a booster at around a year (or at least 2 months from the third dose). Adults were formerly recommended to get the *Pneumovax-23®* at 65 years of age, or earlier if they suffered from any number of chronic diseases (i.e. diabetes, heart or kidney failure, HIV, asthma or chronic smoking.)

The development of *Prevnar13®* (improved from *Prevnar-7*) has resulted in changes in recommendations for adults over 65. In seniors who have not been previously vaccinated, they should receive a *Prevnar-13®* shot first, followed by a *Pneumovax-23®* from 6-12 months later. If they have already received the *Pneumovax-23®*, they should get the *Prevnar-13®* at least a year after their previous pneumonia vaccination.

Healthy People 2020 would like to see 90% pneumococcal vaccination of all seniors over 65. Current pneumococcal vaccination rates, while better than in the past, still hover around 66% or less, depending on the population. Formerly Medicare only covered one pneumococcal shot (except in high-risk individuals), despite the ACIP recommendation to have both. Now both vaccines are reimbursed in the same individual, provided they are given at appropriate ages and intervals. Without insurance, *Pneumovax-23®* costs around $80, while the *Prevnar-13®* costs $170. Double vaccination, with or without reimbursement, certainly beats getting pneumonia, sepsis or even dying. Prevention is always a good investment and all seniors should get vaccinated at 65 years of age (or sooner with some medical conditions.)

SHINGLES: PREVENTABLE
BY VACCINATION

Shingles is an annoying and painful result of reactivation of the Varicella-Zoster Virus (VZV) in the body. Anyone who has had chickenpox (varicella) or has received the varicella vaccination (as most children do) has the potential of developing shingles. About a third of adults will develop this painful condition at some time. The risk increases with age as does the risk of developing postherpetic neuralgia (PHN) as discussed below. There are about 10 cases of shingles/1,000 adults over 60 per year, resulting in about a million cases annually. Around 1% or so will be hospitalized and 96 will die each year, mostly immune-compromised older adults with underlying chronic illnesses or receiving chemotherapy, steroids or other immunosuppressive drugs.

The Varicella-Zoster Virus is highly contagious and most adults born in the U.S. and 40 years of ago or older have had chickenpox (99.5%). As such, they harbor the wild-type VZV in their body. Vaccinated children receive the live attenuated VZV (not the wild-type) and although they also will harbor the Varicella-Zoster Virus, they are less subject to subsequent shingles than children or adults who had the wild-type virus.

Since the virus lives in the nerve roots, shingles manifests itself most often by a characteristic painful, blistering rash that occurs in a dermatome (the specific area on the body surface innervated by a particular nerve). This may occur anywhere on the body, but most often occurs on the trunk. The rash is preceded by several days of itching and tingling pain, followed by the appearance of multiple small blisters in a specific unilateral nerve distribution. These blisters eventually burst, releasing live Varicella-Zoster

Viruses, then subsequently dry up and crust over. Once crusted over, the person is no longer infectious to others.

Shingles can be treated with several anti-viral medications, notably acyclovir, famciclovir or valacyclovir. These can shorten the severity and duration of the rash. Pain relievers are also often required although opioids, if they are used at all, should be restricted to the lowest possible dose for the shortest possible duration. While the blisters persist, the person should avoid contact with pregnant women or adults or children with chronic illness or immunosuppressive medications (i.e. cancer treatment, steroids and some immuno-biological medications for psoriasis, Crohn's disease or rheumatoid arthritis).

Postherpetic neuralgia, a complication of shingles, is particularly annoying since it results in long term pain lasting anywhere from a month to many years after the initial case of shingles. Around 13% of adults over 60 with shingles will develop this debilitating condition. Other serious complications may include painful involvement of the cornea (herpes zoster ophtalmicus) that is heralded by shingles in the nerve that also involves the tip of the nose (a useful clue for clinicians). There can also be rare herpetic complications involving the brain, lungs and liver, all with serious short and long-term consequences.

The appearance of shingles is so characteristic that it can usually be diagnosed without any specific testing. A unilateral, blistering rash, proceeded by pain and tingling, anywhere on the body is usually shingles until proven otherwise. Rare generalized cases can occur in some adults and in children that can be confused with contact dermatitis, drug eruptions, folliculitis or even scabies. These cases can be confirmed with PCR (Polymerase Chain Reaction) testing.

So how can you protect yourself from this painful, annoying and potentially dangerous complication of prior chickenpox or varicella vaccination? The CDC recommends that all adults over 50 (and some younger people with serious health problems) should be vaccinated with Shingrix®. The first dose should be followed by a second one 2 to 6 months later. Protection with Shingrix® exceeds 90%, although it wanes slightly with time. Even those who have received Zostavax® (the previous shingles

vaccine) in the past should be revaccinated. The cost per vial for Shingrix®
is around $172 (according to GoodRx, a very useful app for looking up
local pharmaceutical prices.) Always check with your insurer to verify
coverage for Shingrix® or any other vaccination.

A couple of shots can spare you a lot of potential misery from shingles.

DON'T LET GLAUCOMA ROB
YOU OF YOUR SIGHT

Glaucoma is common, affecting over three million people in the U.S. where it remains the 2nd leading cause of blindness. It is common overseas as well and is reported to affect 14 million people worldwide and is the 3rd leading cause of blindness internationally. Although anyone can get glaucoma, high-risk groups include anyone over 60 years of age, African-Americans over 40, anyone with diabetes and anyone with a family history of glaucoma. Blacks acquire glaucoma 6 to 8 times more often than Whites and anyone with diabetes is twice as likely to get glaucoma as those without that disease. Since diabetes is directly proportional to obesity and Louisiana has over 30% of the population that is obese, the extent of the problem becomes apparent. Because of obesity, around 10% of Louisianans suffer from diabetes (or over 450,000 people in a state of 4.5 million or more than the entire population of Central Louisiana). With the aging population, the problem is only compounded as baby boomers reach 60 years old at a nationwide rate of 10,000 a day.

Glaucoma is complex, with two varieties, closed-angle and open-angle, the latter being the most common. (The "angle" refers to the angle at the junction of the iris and cornea at the edge of the anterior chamber of the eye.) Glaucoma is also subdivided into those that are primary (unknown cause of outflow obstruction) or secondary to some other problem. Open-angle glaucoma results in an increase in intra-ocular pressure that damages the optic nerve, resulting in progressive blindness. Sadly, there may be no symptoms early on in the disease in over 50% of those affected, resulting in silent worsening of the intraocular pressure and increased damage to the optic nerve.

Early diagnosis remains critical to preserving vision. Medicare and many private insurers reimburse glaucoma testing in high-risk groups (African-Americans over 40, anyone over 60, those with diabetes and a family history of glaucoma.) Once diagnosed, it can be treated with various eye drops (usually alpha-2 adrenergic agonists, prostaglandin analogs or beta-blockers). Surgery may also be indicated with different procedures including laser trabeculoplasty, guarded filtration procedure, or possibly tube shunts or ciliodestructive procedures. Details of such treatments and their indications are best left to the ophthalmologist.

The important thing to remember is that glaucoma is frequent and debilitating. Early diagnosis is critical to treatment and that Medicare and many other insurance plans do cover the cost of the screening exam (measurement of intraocular pressure) by an optometrist or ophthalmologist. Complaints of loss of vision, notably missing words when reading, missing stairs when walking, or trouble driving may all be signs of glaucoma. Don't wait until those symptoms appear. Get yourself tested if you are in any of the high-risk groups.

While you're at it, get a flu shot, a herpes zoster vaccine, a TdaP booster, and a pneumococcal vaccine if you are old enough. Prevention is the best medicine, including for the elderly.

SLEEP THAT KNITS THE RAVELED SLEEVE OF CARE

The importance of sleep inspired William Shakespeare with his famous, "Sleep that knits up the raveled sleeve of care" (in Macbeth). In our day and age, sleep still retains its importance for health, both physical and mental.

Inadequate sleep causes the body to increase levels of cortisol, which predisposes to weight gain and diabetes. This is aggravated by the fact that sleep deprivation decreases leptin (the hormone of "fullness") and increases levels of ghrelin (hormone of hunger.) There appears to be a clear association between lack of sleep and weight gain in middle aged and younger subjects. Sleep deprivation also negatively effects wound healing and the immune response, making us more subject to all sorts of infectious diseases.

The greatest negative effects, however, are clearly related to the brain. Lack of sleep causes loss of concentration, impaired memory retention and inattention. It is estimated that twenty percent of bad car accidents are caused by driver fatigue. This amounts to over 250,000 accidents a year involving over 80,000 drivers who have fallen asleep at the wheel. Eighteen hours without sleep is equivalent to a blood alcohol level of 0.05% (the legal limit in Western Europe).

Sleep deprivation effects many critical jobs, among them truck drivers, pilots and doctors. Medical residents now must limit their hours without sleep because of a dangerous increase in errors associated with sleep deprivation. For all students, their performance in fine motor skills drops with less sleep and their emotional responses become more erratic and disinhibited. Most college students report receiving less than 6 hours of nightly sleep and 25% of high school students report falling asleep during class at least once. Worse yet, significant sleep loss increases anxiety, irritability, headaches, depression, suicidal ideation and psychosis, even resulting in hallucinations.

With less than five hours of nightly sleep, the risk of death jumps by 15% (established by a Harvard study). This may be related to an increase in blood pressure and the subsequent increases in heart disease and stroke. With over a third of the adult U.S. population reporting insomnia and associated inadequate sleep, the extent and severity of the problem becomes apparent.

Sleep, like adequate exercise and a healthy diet, should be considered indispensable for young people and adults alike. Although we can sometimes get by with less sleep, consistent sleeplessness can have disastrous short and long-term consequences.

While talking about sleep, I would be remiss to not talk about "Safe Sleep." Safe sleep refers to infants and is geared to reducing the 3,490 infants that die each year from Sudden Infant Death (SIDS), Accidental Suffocation and Strangulation in Bed (ASSB) and "Unknown Causes." Although the number of Sudden Unexpected Infant Deaths (SUID) has decreased over the last two decades (from around 150/100,000 live births to around 80/100,000), largely related to the successful "back to sleep" campaign. Nonetheless, every infant death remains an incredible tragedy, especially if it is preventable.

Some simple steps can reduce the rate of SIDS even further: (1) put infants on their backs (Back to Sleep) (2) Never co-sleep with infants (3) Use a crib with a firm mattress and NO bumpers, blankets, toys or pillows (4) Use light, one-piece sleepers (5) Breastfeed and (6) Never smoke around an infant. These simple steps can reduce the number of sudden infant deaths even more.

So if you are an adult, adolescent or infant, sleep remains a critical component of a healthy life and "Safe Sleep" for infants can actually save their lives as well.

PREP (PRE-EXPOSURE PROPHYLAXIS): A PILL TO PREVENT HIV

Pre-Exposure Prophylaxis (PrEP) is the use of a daily pill, Truvada® (emtricitabine and tenofovir disoproxil) in selected individuals to keep them from contracting HIV. The medication, while very expensive, does prove cost-effective by preventing HIV in some individuals. When taken daily, PrEP reduces the risk of getting HIV by at least 70%.

Truvada® use is not a treatment for HIV as a single drug. In fact, prospective candidates for PrEP must be tested to make sure they do not already have HIV. Only those who are HIV negative and are at high risk for contracting HIV should be considered for PrEP.

One in four sexually active gay and bisexual men (25%) and 1 in 200 sexually active heterosexual adults (0.8%) may be candidates. PrEP may also be indicated in around one in five active drug users (18%). Who are these candidates for PrEP and how are the selected?

First, a PrEP candidate is a HIV negative person who has a HIV positive partner, or multiple partners, or a partner with multiple partners, or a partner of unknown HIV status and has unprotected anal sex or has had a recently documented STD.

Second, PrEP is indicated for those who do not have HIV and who inject drugs and who share needles, or recently underwent a drug rehabilitation treatment (methadone, buprenophine, Suboxone®) or who engage in high risk sexual activity.

Third, PrEP should be used in sexually active heterosexual adults who are HIV negative and have an HIV positive partner, or have multiple partners or a partner having sex with multiple partners of unknown HIV status and have unprotected sex with people who inject drugs or are women who have unprotected sex with bisexual men.

PrEP does not need to be prescribed by specialists, but it does need to go to the appropriate high-risk groups. Despite proven efficacy and established guidelines, PrEP is grossly underutilized. In 2017, only 34% of primary care providers were aware of the existence of PrEP. Even those who do have access to PrEP do not always use it.

Once established, a prospective candidate must be tested for HIV. If positive, the person is not a PrEP candidate, but should be referred for appropriate treatment of HIV. If negative, the provider must establish if the person is a high risk individual. If high risk and HIV negative, a baseline blood test is obtained to establish normal kidney function. If normal, health care providers need to proceed with inquiries about insurance status with the hopes of entering the person in a payment assistance program. Finally, a prescription can be written and the person safely started on Truvada®.

As mentioned, correct use of PrEP can reduce the occurrence of HIV by anywhere from 70 to 90%. Use of PrEP does not decrease the need for safe needle usage and reduction of high-risk sexual activity. We cannot allow ignorance of PrEP or underutilization to negatively affect reducing infectious risks in these high-risk groups.

Due to the paucity of PrEP providers in some areas of the state, a system of Tele-PrEP has been established to assure access. Trained APRN (advanced practice nurses) will prescribe PrEP after interviews and review of appropriate lab results.

Besides PrEP, the other pillars of HIV reduction include widespread HIV testing, encouraging adherence to HIV treatment and universal viral suppression. These, plus systematic condom use and needle exchange programs should help achieve significant reductions in the HIV epidemic.

PROSTATE SPECIFIC ANTIGEN (PSA), PROSTATE CANCER AND LONGEVITY

Affecting millions of men (with around 150,000 new cases a year), prostate cancer once defied early diagnosis and almost always presented with late stage disease, often metastatic locally or at a distance, with a corresponding poor prognosis. Even today, about 26,000 men die each year in the U.S, from prostate cancer. Age-adjusted deaths from prostate cancer in 1986 were 34.9/100,000. That same year, PSA (Prostate Specific Antigen) was invented by Richard Albin as a lab test to detect early prostate cancer by means of a simple blood test. When first introduced, it promised to revolutionize the detection and treatment of prostate cancer and presumably greatly reduce deaths from that disease. New diagnoses did increase from 119/100,000 in 1986 to a high of 180.3/100.00 in 2001, dropping to a low of 96.1/100,000 by 2014.

PSA allowed earlier detection of prostate cancer and initiated an era of earlier diagnosis and treatment, either surgical or radiological or some combination of the two. While drops in death rates have occurred (from 34.9/100,000 in 1986 to 19.1/100,000 in 2014) substantial prolongation of life remained elusive. While some morbidity associated with advanced prostate cancer also decreased, there was no significant increase in life expectancy, just fewer deaths from prostate cancer itself.

With subsequent research, it became clear that aggressive treatment did not benefit all men and that most would die from causes other than prostate cancer. The expression became "you died with prostate cancer, but not from prostate cancer." What's more, the treatments carried significant possible side effects which included persistent urinary incontinence and impotence, not to mention considerable medical costs. Richard J. Albin, the inventor of the PSA test even said that use of his test was "a profit-driven public health disaster."

It used to be recommended that all men be tested with a PSA at age 50 (or earlier with a family history of prostate cancer). The pendulum of recommendations from the USPTF (United States Preventive Task Force) swung back a couple of years ago, however, to a far more conservative stance. Doctors are now encouraged not to do systematic PSA testing except when the patient presents with signs of outlet obstruction (difficulty urinating related to prostatic hypertrophy) and then only after a one-on-one discussion about the risk and benefits of a diagnosis of prostate cancer. Biannual testing in African-Americans over 50 may be justified because of high rates of prostate cancer in that group. The same holds true for those with a significant family history of prostate cancer. PSA testing after 70 years of age is not recommended at all.

As mentioned, deaths from prostate cancer declined for decades after the advent of PSA (34.9/100,000 in 1986 to 19.1/100,000 in 2014). As in the pre-PSA past, however, late diagnosis has again became a reality, with associated significant morbidity and mortality. While most men with prostate cancer die "with the disease and not because of it," those with advanced disease still die from prostate cancer albeit at a reduced rate from past decades.

So what should be done? Early testing (and better treatments) may have yielded a substantial reduction in deaths, but no prolongation of life. Doing nothing, however, does not seem justified. At the present, a talk with your doctor about urinary symptoms and a one-on-one discussion about risks and benefits of diagnosis and non-diagnosis of prostate cancer is justified.

This ongoing debate, not unlike that associated with the use of mammograms, underlines the fact that all tests and all treatments must have a positive benefit to risk ratio. With additional data collection and analysis, we should be able to better define those who will benefit from the use of PSA versus those for whom its use will only add cost and inconvenience with no added years of life. In the end, the doctors must still follow the cardinal rule of medicine, "*primum non nocere*" (first, do no harm). Patients should make informed decisions based on facts and not emotions.

WELL-AHEAD AND WELL SPOTS

The Louisiana Department of Health and Hospitals, under the previous direction of Secretary Kathy Kliebert and the current direction of Dr. Rebecca Gee, inaugurated a program to enlist and encourage healthy initiatives among diverse prospective partners. The justification for such a move comes from a sincere desire to improve the health outcomes of our citizens and the health statistics for Louisiana, which currently ranks 49/50 among states (America's Health Rankings 2017).

Louisiana ranks particularly poorly for smoking, obesity, infant mortality, sexually transmitted diseases (including HIV/AIDS), premature deaths and preventable hospitalizations. This makes improving health outcomes a critical priority for the state. Real people suffer from real, preventable diseases and collaborative approaches to health initiatives prove the most successful.

So what is WELL-AHEAD? WELL-AHEAD is a statewide Louisiana program that hopes to encourage the development of many WELL SPOTS scattered throughout the state. Different entities, whether they are individuals, childcare centers, schools, colleges and universities, hospitals, restaurants, or other worksites and businesses, must each satisfy a specific number of criteria to achieve WELL SPOT designation. These criteria vary from entity to entity, but all must be tobacco-free (not just smoke-free). Most other entities must also be "Breastfeeding Friendly" and adhere to the 5-2-1-0 program (5 fruits and vegetables, less than 2 hours screen time, 1 hour of physical activity and 0 sweetened beverages per day.)

Other criteria for institutions include completion of the 7 steps of the LA Business Group on Health toolkit, healthy vending choices and administrative buy-in for the WELL SPOT initiative. Birthing hospitals must be designated as GIFT hospitals (related to aggressive plans to promote breast feeding), or "Baby Friendly," a more stringent program with the same goal. Restaurants need to not only offer healthy food choices (including Kids LiveWell Program suggestions), but also have ServSafe trained food and beverage handlers, all in a tobacco-free environment.

When entities achieve their WELL SPOT designation, they will be acknowledged and celebrated both regionally and statewide. Depending on the number of criteria met, an entity is designated as achieving Level Three, Two or One (the highest.) While such recognition provides a certain incentive, the real motivation and validation will be a progressive increase in Louisiana's health rankings.

By enlisting the help and cooperation of non-governmental groups, health should become the focus not only of a few healthcare-related professionals, but of society as a whole. The real beneficiaries of such an improvement, so important to public health providers, are the citizens of Louisiana who will individually (and collectively) lead longer and healthier lives.

For more information, please consult: http://www.dhh.louisiana.gov/index.cfm/page/1833/n/394

MASS SHOOTINGS: A PUBLIC HEALTH MENACE

Public Health deals with problems of groups, unlike regular healthcare providers who concentrate on individual cases. When a problem such as opioid abuse reaches epidemic proportions, Public Health seeks ways to mitigate the issue and prevent it from happening. In fact, Public Health usually focuses on preventive measures rather than on individual treatments (with some exceptions, of course.)

One such public health issue rises to the surface repeatedly with catastrophic consequences: mass shootings. Not a month goes by that we are not confronted by the horrific images of victims of a mass shooting, often in school settings. Although such events do seem to occur sporadically in other countries, nothing approaches the scope and magnitude of this problem in the United States.

There have been numerous attempts to identify the reasons for this epidemic, which has been attributed to mental health issues, violent video games, criminality and other explanations. The fact is that the disproportionate number of U.S. mass shootings is directly proportional to the number of guns per capita. The U.S. population is less than 5% of the world's total, yet we boast 42% of the world's gun ownerships. We also account for over 30% of the mass shootings.

Americans do not appear to suffer from any unusually elevated percentage of people suffering from mental health problems. Nor are we more prone to criminality (despite our disproportionate incarceration rates.) Only 4% of gun-related deaths were related to mental health problems. And Americans watch about the same amount of violent video games as in other developed countries.

What it comes down to is that we are a nation awash in firearms, some of which have no other purpose than mass destruction (i.e. assault rifles). Protecting the right to bear arms appears to be a national obsession. Yet it comes with a huge price tag. How many avoidable school shootings can we tolerate as a society? Should we tolerate even one? It has been suggested that our persistent indifference to the slaughter of innocents represents a moral Rubicon that we crossed after the massacre at Sandy Hook Elementary without weighing or appreciating the long-term consequences. Doing nothing at that time has become the pattern for subsequent events with mind-numbing regularity.

Public Health deals with prevention and the road to prevention appears to be abundantly clear in the case of mass shootings if we are willing to pursue it. Common sense and morality should dictate policy, not a visceral protection of an ill-defined right to bear arms that is only recognized by a handful of countries around the world. There is clearly a cost/benefit ratio that should be dispassionately considered.

Can we stop isolated lunatics from assaulting their fellow citizens? Perhaps not, but we can certainly decrease the senseless carnage. Thoughtful gun control appears to be the only solution. If we insist on swimming in a sea of guns, then we must be willing to drown in continued massacres of the innocents in an endless succession of school shootings and other slaughters.

ABOUT THE AUTHOR

Dr. David J. Holcombe was born in San Francisco, California in 1949 and raised in the East Bay. He attended the U. of California at Davis (BSA 1971) and went on to study at the Institute of Food and Agricultural Sciences at the U. of Florida in Gainesville (MSA 1975). He subsequently attended the Catholic U. of Louvain in Brussels, Belgium, where he received his M.D. Summa Cum Laude in 1981.

Returning to the U.S. with his charming Belgian wife and the first of four sons, he completed a residency in internal medicine at a Johns-Hopkins affiliated clinic in Baltimore, Maryland. He and his family subsequently moved to Alexandria, Louisiana in 1986, where he worked 20 years as an internist with a busy multi-specialty clinic. He then assumed a regional position in public health in 2007.

During his years of medical study, he continued to paint, write and folk dance, all very non-medical passions. He self-published two volumes of short stories, four volumes of plays, one volume of medical articles (most of which previously appeared in two regional publications, *CenLA Focus* and *Visible Horizon*), and a hybrid publication of scientific articles and corresponding original plays (*Public Health Onstage*).

He has served on the board of Spectral Sisters Productions, a local developmental theatre company for 14 years. His artwork has been accepted in many juried art shows both locally and regionally and his paintings are in collections all over the U.S. and abroad. He volunteers as a Civil Surgeon for Community Health Worx (a local free clinic), helps with the PrEP Clinic at the Central Louisiana AIDS Support

Services and serves on an Institutional Review Board among other charitable activities. He is sometimes referred to as the "Chekhov on the Bayou."

Both he and his wife, Nicole, are committed to making Central Louisiana a better place through continuous social capital building.

Printed in the United States
By Bookmasters